W9-BVR-028

Just What the Doctor Ordered

Just What the Doctor Ordered

THE INSIDER'S GUIDE TO GETTING INTO MEDICAL SCHOOL IN CANADA

Christine Fader

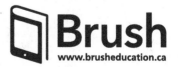

www.brusheducation.ca

Copyright © 2018 Christine Fader

18 19 20 21 22 5 4 3 2 1

Printed and manufactured in Canada

Thank you for buying this book and for not copying, scanning, or distributing any part of it without permission. By respecting the spirit as well as the letter of copyright, you support authors and publishers, allowing them to continue to create and distribute the books you value.

Excerpts from this publication may be reproduced under licence from Access Copyright, or with the express written permission of Brush Education Inc., or under licence from a collective management organization in your territory. All rights are otherwise reserved, and no part of this publication may be reproduced, stored in a retrieval system, or transmitted in any form or by any means, electronic, mechanical, photocopying, digital copying, scanning, recording, or otherwise, except as specifically authorized.

Brush Education Inc.

www.brusheducation.ca

contact@brusheducation.ca

Cover design: Dean Pickup; cover image (doctor's pocket) from Dreamstime.com: Jakgapong Pengjank

Interior design: Carol Dragich, Dragich Design

Library and Archives Canada Cataloguing in Publication

Fader, Christine, 1969-, author
    Just what the doctor ordered : the insider's guide to getting into medical school in Canada / Christine Fader.

Issued in print and electronic formats.

ISBN 978-1-55059-770-7 (softcover).—ISBN 978-1-55059-771-4 (PDF).—ISBN 978-1-55059-772-1 (Kindle).—ISBN 978-1-55059-773-8 (EPUB).

    1. Medical colleges—Canada—Entrance requirements. 2. Medical colleges—Canada—Admission. 3. Medical colleges—Canada. I. Title.

R838.4.F33 2018   610.71'171   C2018-904168-4
                                         C2018-904169-2

We acknowledge the support of the Government of Canada
Nous reconnaissons l'appui du gouvernement du Canada | Canada

Contents

Introduction

"I got in!"

These are three of my favourite words, and I am fortunate to hear them quite regularly from the medical-school applicants I work with directly. I wish I could hear them even more than I already do. This is part of what has led me to write this resource: the idea that more students might benefit from the information, perspectives, and strategies that other applicants to medical school have found useful.

I hope this resource gives support and encouragement to your dreams of becoming a physician, and concrete ideas and strategies for success in a challenging process. I hope it will, in some small way, help you be the next one to say: I got in!

Why this resource?

If you're reading this resource, you are likely already aware of how challenging the process of admission to a Canadian medical school can be. If you are like many applicants, you may have already tried applying on your own, without success.

You are not alone. Most medical-school applicants I see have extremely high grade point averages, not to mention extracurricular and community activities galore. They tend to apply to many medical schools, yet receive only one or two interviews—if any. Many of the accomplished students who have sought my help are on their second or third application attempt.

How can this be?

I believe part of the answer lies in numbers. There are ninety-six universities in Canada with a total student population of about 1.8 million. Not every student hopes to become a physician, of course, but take a moment to think about how many students you know in high school or university who are thinking about medical school. When I worked at orientation fairs for incoming students to first-year university, the question I got most from students and parents was: Can you tell me what courses we need to get into medical school?

So, there are potentially lots of interested students. We have limited numbers of medical schools in Canada and limited numbers of spots available at each school. This means that the posted "minimum requirements" from medical schools don't necessarily reflect the reality of a successful application in Canada.

When I visited a Caribbean medical school several years ago, I spent a week with several premedical advisors from the United States. As the only Canadian advisor, I was startled to hear some of the statistics that my American counterparts told me represented their students: grade point averages in the low 2s (out of 4), and entrance exam scores far lower than any I had seen in my daily work at a Canadian university.

I thought to myself: If the students I worked with had similar statistics, I could understand why they didn't receive offers of admission. But their statistics were much better—even among students who were applying to Caribbean medical schools because they felt they couldn't compete with applicants to Canadian medical schools.

The students I have seen in the last twenty years have, by an overwhelming majority, strong academics and good test scores, and contribute enthusiastically, consistently, and broadly in their larger communities. Yet, less than fourteen percent of applicants to medical school received offers in 2015–2016 in Ontario.[1] This percentage appears to be similar across Canada.

In my experience, most medical-school hopefuls—whether they are in high school or university—are used to setting difficult goals and achieving them. The goal of admission to medical school, or the perceived "failure" to achieve it (if you have applied before), can present the biggest challenge you have ever faced. I have seen this challenge erode the confidence of the most stellar students, but I have also seen those students and many others persevere and succeed.

Why this author?
I'd like to tell you a bit about why I think I can help.

Over the last twenty years working as a career advisor at a Canadian university, I have worked with thousands of students, from first-year undergraduates to PhD candidates, in diverse degree programs from fine arts to engineering physics. My work has involved helping undergraduate and graduate students explore career options, consider related degree decisions, strategize about further education, search for jobs, and improve their career-development knowledge and skills.

During this time—in my university job and, since 2007, in my private practice—I have also worked with thousands of students hoping to become physicians. I have an "insider" perspective on the health sector from a wide range of experience. For example, for eight years, I volunteered as a community member on a medical-school admissions committee, where I reviewed applications and interviewed candidates. I was not involved in selecting candidates, and I do not speak for medical schools or their selection criteria (particularly since admissions procedures have evolved since my committee work), but I did screen many candidates and came to recognize qualities that, in my judgement, made some candidates stand out. I have also developed and delivered hundreds of workshops on applying to, and interviewing for, medical school and residency programs, and have spent eighteen years working with final-year medical students and international medical graduates applying to residency programs.

So, I offer you:

- experience as someone who has read thousands of medical-school applications and coached thousands of students through application strategies and medical-school interviews (in my private practice, I have given personalized coaching to a hundred or so students—all, except one, have succeeded in getting accepted to medical school)
- knowledge of the processes, terminology, and challenges of medical school and residency programs
- stories of applicants who have struggled and ultimately succeeded in their goals
- twenty years of coaching students to medical school and residency placements
- career-counselling techniques to help you present yourself as an informed and focused applicant, and to develop crucial backup plans

And I offer you the experience of hundreds of thousands of hours working with students just like you.

However, I want you to be skeptical of any secondhand source (and that includes me and a long list of others: medical students, doctors, advisors, guidance counsellors, parents, and helpful books and friends). Only the medical schools themselves, in the year that you plan to apply, have the most current and accurate information or interpretation of a given "rule." Be wary of people or sources (websites, campus clubs, mentoring groups) that make definitive statements about "rules": the rules come from processes that continually evolve. Every "expert" (including me) is filtering information through their own lens. We are merely interpreters and **not** the source. Make sure that you are getting the information that **you** need and can trust. That means **always** validate what you hear, read, see, or suspect from **the source**—in other words, from the people who will take your application money and decide your future in their program.

To be clear: **the source is each medical school in the year you plan to apply.**

Repeat this to yourself! Chant it whenever you are tempted to take shortcuts and assume that someone else knows what they are talking about.

For example, your question might be, Does my human geography course count as a humanities prerequisite for medical school? The "expert" answer of a secondhand source is always: Blah, blah, blah, blah, blah. They might sound very sure of themselves as they answer your question—but what you should hear, especially with a question that asks them to interpret what a medical school wants, is blah, blah, blah, blah, blah.

You can listen to what the person says, and think of it as possibly true, but always remember it is only one perspective. You need to verify the information directly from the medical school itself. Yes, this means more work for you, but it is really important work to do. Pretend a patient's life is at stake, because it is: you are the patient in this case.

This resource and other people will help you get information and ideas that can be very useful in your process. You can incorporate some of those views and advice (and mine) into your strategy. But always, *always* remember that what is true for them, and true for now, might not be true for you or true when you apply.

I wrote this resource less as a "do this, do that" manual and more as a "think about this, think about that" strategy tool. This is my biggest gift to you: a strategy to find your own "insider" perspective, which, in my experience, has produced the most confident and competent applicants in the end.

Why start in high school?

While my primary client base is university and postgraduate students, I do work with some high school students. I wanted to include them in this book because I believe that starting earlier in the process (without overly stressing our students) can be a helpful way to pace out an application to medical school, review additional career options, and ultimately have a less difficult and more successful application process, if and when the time comes around. This resource has a specific chapter for high school students, but also many additional strategy suggestions throughout.

Why include parents?

In my experience, parents and other supporters often play a large and vital part in encouraging medical-school hopefuls, so that's why I have included a chapter for them in this resource. If you are a parent, or have a parent or supporter who is aware of your medical-school hopes, take a look at chapter 17. I hope it gives parents strategies to help support students embarking on this process, as well as some information about what students might be facing as they do so.

If you are a student with well-meaning parents or supporters, I suggest leaving that chapter lying casually open somewhere, in a place they might trip over it. They want to help you and this might be a good start.

Note
1. Vanessa Milne, Christopher Doig, Irfan Dhalla, "Less Science, More Diversity: How Canadian Medical School Admissions Are Changing," *HealthyDebate.ca*, December 25, 2015, http://healthydebate.ca/2015/12/topic/canadian-medical-schools-admissions.

PART I

GETTING READY

*Read this section if you are in high school, early
university, or new to the application process.*

1

How do you become a doctor?

Don't skip this chapter!

Whether you've arrived at the goal of becoming a doctor only
recently, or have been dreaming about it since you first played Oper-
ation as a child, you need to know the steps involved in actually
achieving this goal. Even if you think you know, it's important to be
sure you *really know*.

It can be such a challenge getting into medical school that students and families often focus only on the getting-in part, and not
on what happens afterwards. In my experience, many candidates for
medical school are only vaguely aware, or not at all informed, about
the full path to becoming a fully licensed physician—how long it
takes, the competitive processes involved, and how much it can cost.

Knowing this information feeds into your ability to come across
as an informed candidate—someone who knows the good, bad, and
ugly about becoming a physician in Canada. This information can
also help you pace yourself from a mental- and physical-wellness
perspective: this is a long and arduous road, and knowing what's
ahead can help you prepare.

Perhaps the first thing to clarify is the difference between "doctor"
and "doctor" and "doctor." You are probably aware that there are
several types of professionals in the workplace with the title "doctor." But, which doctors went through medical school and which

3

didn't? Even if you have friends or family who have gone to university or become doctors, it can be a little mysterious. In addition, many educators assume everyone understands these differences—it can be embarrassing to ask questions about it, if everyone else seems already to know the deal.

MD versus PhD: What's the difference?

PhD doctors

University students encounter this type of doctor among their professors. Doctors with PhDs usually don't work with patients (except, perhaps, in a research capacity). Professors receive the title "doctor" after they finish their doctor of philosophy (PhD). A PhD can be in virtually any subject. For example, I have friends with PhDs in English, German, civil engineering, and occupational therapy. If you're familiar with the television show *The Big Bang Theory*, you may recall that Sheldon (theoretical physics), Leonard (experimental physics), Raj (astrophysics), Amy (neurobiology), and Bernadette (microbiology) all hold PhDs. They are all called "doctor," but none of them went to medical school.

If you're considering medicine because you love school, enjoy going in-depth on a topic, or just plain love learning, a PhD might be an additional or alternate career option for you. People with PhDs work in universities as professors (usually doing a combination of research, teaching, and administration), in research institutes, for pharmaceutical companies, in government, and more.

Check out PhD.org for more information about this type of doctor.

Clinician doctors

In North America, we call a dentist Dr. So-and-so. We call an optometrist Dr. So-and-so. It's the same with chiropractors, chiropodists, naturopathic doctors, and clinical psychologists, just to name a few. All of these kinds of doctors work with patients, but they didn't go to medical school.

These professionals either have a specific degree that governs their focus (e.g., doctor of dentistry, doctor of optometry, doctor of chiropody) or a combination of academic and clinical education (e.g., a PhD in clinical psychology) that licences them to work with patients. They are highly trained in programs that teach specific skills. Learners practise in their field under supervision, and clinicians are governed by regulations and rules of professional practice that protect both clinicians and patients. These people are all doctors, but they are not physicians in the way that we are talking about in this resource.

Students applying to medical school often really want to work with patients, which might make a variety of clinical roles a good fit. Chapter 3 discusses some clinical roles that you might want to consider. A great thing to ask yourself as you apply to medical school is, Why become a physician and not one of these other "doctor" options?

Medical doctors

Now we arrive at the type of doctor this book discusses. The degree you'll do if you go to medical school in Canada is a doctor of medicine (MD). In the United States, there is also something called a doctor of osteopathy (DO), which is very common there and can be an alternate to a traditional MD for students in that country. In England, where you generally enter medical school right after high school, you get a bachelor of medicine (MB).

In Canada, you need to do part or all of an undergraduate degree before you start medical school. After you get an MD, you must complete additional training before you can legally work as a physician (see *Figure 1*).

Medical school in Canada is considered "undergraduate medical education." This seems confusing, since you can't enter medical school until you have completed part or all of an undergraduate degree. So, let's clarify: medical school is "undergraduate" in the sense that you are at the first stage of becoming a physician. "Postgraduate" medical education (or residency) occurs after you complete an MD and before you're allowed to practise medicine with a license.

Medical school in Canada usually takes four years. Some schools offer a three-year option (this option simply compresses content so that summers are spent at school). These programs offer the same degree at the end, so the choice is really about your personal timelines and preferences.

UNDERGRADUATE DEGREE

Complete at least three years of undergraduate study. (Some medical schools require a complete undergraduate degree.) Note that some candidates also complete one or more graduate degrees.

MEDICAL SCHOOL

Complete three or four years of study (this varies by medical school) to achieve a medical degree (MD). (An MD does not make you a licensed physician.)
Pass the Medical Council of Canada Qualifying Exam Part I.
Apply to residency programs. (This happens during the final year of medical school and is a competitive process.)
Match to a residency program.

RESIDENCY

Complete two to seven years of training (this varies by specialty) and pass required evaluations.

QUALIFYING EXAMS

Pass the Medical Council of Canada Qualifying Exam Part II (or an approved equivalent).
Pass residency-certification exams (or approved equivalents). (The certifying authority varies by residency. The certifying authorities in Canada include the Royal College of Physicians and Surgeons of Canada, the College of Family Physicians of Canada, and the Collège des médecins du Québec.)
Note that some people do fellowships, or pursue specialties that require additional training and qualifying exams.

PHYSICIAN

Receive a license to practise. (This is awarded at the discretion of provincial and territorial regulators—for example, the College of Physicians and Surgeons of Ontario, the College of Physicians and Surgeons of British Columbia, and so on.)

Figure 1. The (usual) path to becoming a physician in Canada

It is important to note the time commitment required. The shortest possible path to becoming a physician tends to be as follows:

- get accepted at a school that will admit you after three years of undergraduate courses (three years)
- finish a three-year MD at a school that offers it (three years)
- do a family medicine residency (two years)

Total time commitment(shortest possible) = 3 + 3 + 2 = 8 years

So you could be a physician eight years after completing high school. Very speedy. It's possible, but it's definitely not typical.

At the opposite end of the spectrum is a friend of mine. She did a four-year undergraduate degree and applied to medical school in her final year. She didn't get accepted to medical school, but she did get accepted to a research master's program. She completed that degree in two years and reapplied to medical school in her final year. She then completed a four-year medical degree and got accepted into residency training for neurosurgery. That was a six-year residency, at the end of which she got accepted in a one-year pediatric neurosurgery fellowship for specialized training.

Total time commitment (real-life example) = 4 + 2 + 4 + 6 + 1 = 17 years

She was in her midthirties before she started her "real" job. As I said, she is a bit of an extreme example.

However, most medical-school applicants complete at least a full undergraduate degree (if not more) before gaining admission to medical school. Most people complete their MD in four years. Most residency training takes two to four years. That means most people can expect to spend at least ten to twelve years after high school in becoming a fully licensed physician.

INSIDER INSIGHT
When you are being assessed as an applicant, the people reviewing your scores, reading your application, and interviewing you have in mind the time it takes to become a physician. They wonder: Do you really understand the time commitment involved in getting educated for this career? Do you realize that you may be putting off—for an extended period—things like having a family, buying property, and living in one place?

In Canada in 2018, there was at least one exception to this typical time commitment. Queen's University and Queen's Medical School now admits up to ten students to medical school immediately after high school. This program is called Queen's University Accelerated Route to Medical School (QuARMS). Visit the QuARMS website for more information (use *QuARMS* as the search term in your browser). Given how many years it takes the average person to become a fully licensed physician, I wonder if this unique Queen's program is a trend that will spread.

In medical school, you will be exposed to a variety of career areas within medicine.

Fields of work within medicine are loosely divided into two categories: medical specialties and surgical specialties. Medical specialties focus on training in medical practices and techniques, and include disciplines such as family medicine, general internal medicine, psychiatry, pediatrics, emergency medicine, hematology, neurology, and more. Surgical specialties focus on training in surgical techniques and practices, and include disciplines such as general surgery, cardiac surgery, neurosurgery, and orthopaedic surgery, and also disciplines that have significant surgical elements such as anesthesiology, obstetrics and gynecology, urology, ophthalmology, otolaryngology, and more.

For more information about medical specialties, consider the following helpful resources: *How to Choose a Medical Specialty* by Anita D. Taylor (2016), and the specialty profiles on the website of the Canadian Medical Association (use *specialty profiles* and *Canadian Medical Association* as the search terms in your browser).

You will be required to do supervised work in a hospital ("clinical rotations") in a variety of medical specialties (e.g., family medicine, pediatrics, psychiatry) and surgical specialties (e.g., general surgery, obstetrics and gynecology, anesthesiology). You will also complete "electives" at your own medical school's hospital, or other hospitals around the country, to practise skills and make contacts within fields that you think you might want to pursue. During rotations and electives, you will be supervised by senior medical students, residents, and attending physicians. You will work with other members of the health-care team, including nurses, therapists, social workers, orderlies, and administrators. You will take "call" shifts where you are the medical student "on call," who is responsible for dealing with any issues (appropriate to your level) that arise on the hospital ward or floor to which you've been assigned.

At some medical schools, you will begin having intensive contact with patients right from the beginning of your degree. At others, the first couple of years will have a more basic-science focus before introducing you to intensive clinical work.

As you move through medical school, you will gain insights into your own preferences, affinities, and skills. You'll likely attend brown-bag lunches hosted by physicians in particular specialties, so you can learn more about their daily work and careers. You may even be part of a student interest group for a particular discipline (e.g., a urology interest group or a general internal medicine interest group). These experiences help you refine your own career interests, and will give you opportunities to connect with professionals in those fields.

About clerkship

Towards the end of medical school, you will enter what is called "clerkship." This involves intensive rotations and electives in hospitals, and is an opportunity to develop evidence to showcase when you apply to residency, during your final year.

You don't normally have much choice about rotations. You are required to complete a certain number of weeks in a prescribed set of disciplines (e.g., family medicine, general surgery). There may be specialties you really don't care for and others you love. You might find your passion or niche, or you might find nothing that really grabs you. The goal is to see where your skills and personality fit, and in what cultures and disciplines you feel most comfortable.

You will also arrange, in conjunction with your medical school, "elective" time. These are blocks of time (usually a few weeks) when you work in specialties and locations that are of potential interest to you for residency. These electives can take place at any medical school in Canada, so you will be travelling to, and living in, a variety of locations during this time. You might be doing a dermatology elective at the University of Toronto for a few weeks, and then a radiology elective at the University of Calgary.

There is some strategy involved in picking your electives, which your medical school will likely help coach you through. Residency programs review your electives when you apply, to see if you have demonstrated interest in the discipline involved in their program (e.g., a residency program in cardiac surgery might look for an elective in cardiac surgery), possibly even at their location (e.g., the University of Manitoba).

About applying for residency

Residency applications are competitive, and they are centralized in Canada through a system called the Canadian Residency Match Service (CaRMS).

Final-year medical students apply to residency programs across the country (and sometimes outside Canada) through the CaRMS website by November of their final year. Residency applications involve a variety of components, such as a curriculum vitae (CV) and letters of reference, and are reviewed by program directors at medical schools across Canada. The program directors decide whom to interview, and interviews often take place in the winter of the final year of medical school. You may spend many weeks travelling around the country to interviews, if you have applied broadly. After interviews, program directors across the country post their lists of top applicants via the CaRMS system, and students across the country post the programs they would like to attend, ranked in order of preference. Then, usually in early March, comes "Match Day." Every medical student's future seems to pivot on this day. Will they get accepted to the residency program (and, with luck, location) of their choice? Will they get accepted at all? Rest assured, the answer is overwhelmingly yes.

About residency

Once students are accepted to a residency program, they move (depending on the location of their residency) and begin life with the letters *MD* after their names. However, they still require a great deal of supervision, because they are not yet fully licensed physicians.

First-year residents are supervised by attending physicians (fully licensed physicians) and more-senior residents as they learn the specialized skills required in their chosen disciplines. As mentioned before, completing a residency takes more or less time, depending on the specialty. In addition, many residents choose to subspecialize (move to a more specific area within their broader discipline—for example, from general internal medicine to cardiology or hematology) or do a fellowship, which adds time to their training.

The good news is that residents are working in hospitals while they study (they also have course work to complete), they're addressed as "doctor" (having earned their MD), and they are being paid a salary. They also tend to work long hours, so many residents comment that the hourly wage is best not calculated.

For more information about residency, visit the website of the Professional Association of Residents of Ontario (PARO) or other provincial residency websites.

Qualifying exams, licensure, certification

The exams that lead to full licensure to practise medicine in Canada mostly take place toward the end of residency or within twenty months of residency completion.

Medical Council of Canada

Before someone can practise medicine in Canada, they must be granted the Licentiate of the Medical Council of Canada (LMCC), which involves two exams: the Medical Council of Canada Qualifying Exam Part I and Part II (MCCQE Part I and MCCQE Part II). Graduates of medical school complete the MCCQE Part I (a written exam). Residents or residency graduates complete the MCCQE Part II (an objective structured clinical exam, or OSCE). If you're thinking of attending a medical school outside Canada, and you want to practise in Canada, you should take particular note of the LMCC requirements, which are covered in chapter 19.

United States Medical Licensing Exams

Similar to Canada, the United States conducts examinations to grant licenses for physicians to practise in the US. Some Canadian and international medical graduates choose to pursue this option. Their exams are called the United States Medical Licensing Examinations (USMLEs).

Royal College of Physicians and Surgeons of Canada, and other certification authorities

Residents or residency graduates must receive certification through the Royal College of Physicians and Surgeons of Canada, the College of Family Physicians of Canada, or the Collège des médecins du Québec (the certifying authority depends on the residency). Certification can involve written exams and OSCEs.

International Medical Graduates (IMGs)

Some Canadian students choose to attend medical school in other countries and want to return to Canada to practise. Some physicians who have been fully trained elsewhere emigrate to Canada. These students and physicians are considered international medical graduates (IMGs). Chapter 19 has more information about this category of applicant.

2

Why is it so hard to get in?

Hardly a day goes by in Canada that we aren't struck by the tensions our health-care system faces. We hear about people who can't find a family doctor, delays for elective surgeries, long wait times to see specialists, overloaded emergency departments and "hallway" care, and medical residents working twenty-four-hour-plus shifts.

It seems obvious that we need more doctors—right? Our hospitals and clinics appear to be bursting at the seams.

So, if we need more doctors, why is it so difficult to get into medical school in Canada? The answer is more complicated and layered than it might appear on the surface. Unfortunately, the burden of that complicated answer often falls on students' shoulders. Parents aren't always completely familiar with the current challenges faced by students today in getting into medical school—even if they are physicians themselves.

This chapter describes some of the factors I have noted over my years of working in this field, which help explain why getting into medical school is so challenging.

Of course, a few students get into medical school on their first attempt. But they are a small minority. Most very qualified students don't know the challenges until they are unsuccessful the first time.

That "failure"—which is really just a normal reality of this process—can be very troubling to them and their families. It might be the first time they have ever failed to achieve a goal that they've set.

That's when I see them in my office, confidence shaken. That's what this resource aims to prevent.

Number of students

I have a German friend who is always astonished about how much work I do with medical-school hopefuls. "It seems as if everyone in Canada wants to be a doctor," she has remarked, somewhat bewildered. Indeed, it must seem that way to Canadian medical-school hopefuls, too.

The numbers say that more and more Canadian students are applying to medical school. For example, applications to medical schools in Ontario (the province with the largest number of medical schools) has increased by thirty percent since 2000.[1]

Okay, so lots of students want to be doctors. Surely, we have enough spots to accommodate them?

Hmmm, let's see.

Number of schools

We currently have 17 medical schools in Canada. Compare that with 143 in the United States and nearly 50 in the Caribbean. In 2017, the 17 schools in Canada received approximately forty thousand applications.[2]

Of Canada's 17 medical schools, 12 are English-language only, 3 (in Quebec) are French-language only, and 2 (McGill and the University of Ottawa) offer programs in both English and French. So, if you're a student wanting to study only in English, your application options reduce from 17 to 14. If you're a student wanting to study only in French, you have only 5 places to apply.

These "odds" are partly why it can be so difficult to get into a program. Because of this, students often apply at multiple locations, regardless of their geographic or institutional preferences.

Class sizes

Some schools (e.g., the University of Toronto) have a large number of spots. Others (e.g., the Northern Ontario School of Medicine) have fewer. These institutional numbers are connected to the size of each university, the amount of funding their program gets, faculty available to teach medical students, lab and classroom space, the number of preceptors available in local hospitals to supervise final-year students, and more.

Occasionally, these numbers increase slightly, but they don't increase exponentially, because of all the other factors I mentioned above, which don't change at the same time. Therefore, even if medical schools were suddenly given permission and money from the government or other benefactors to double their class sizes, the other institutional constraints would mean they couldn't accommodate the growth.

So, medical-school classes are not going to suddenly expand so that everyone who wants to be a doctor can get in. They have expanded some, though—and, in Ontario, this has more or less kept pace with the growth in applicants since 2000. At first glance, by the numbers, the "odds" of getting in should be roughly the same as they were in 2000.

Like many statistics, the numbers oversimplify a complex situation. Based on my observations and experiences with students over the past twenty years, other factors make getting accepted more difficult now than ever before.

Eligibility

Perhaps it's eligibility that makes things more challenging? Not everyone is eligible to apply to every medical school in Canada.

If you are an Ontario resident, you can theoretically apply to all six Ontario medical schools—not bad odds.

Most provinces outside Ontario reserve the majority of their spots for residents of that province. This gives students in those provinces a fair chance at the minimal options they have in their region. It's also often seen as a way to attract applicants who are already established and committed to a province in the hope that they will practise in that province, once they are trained.

There are sometimes a small number of spots for Ontario students at schools in other provinces. The number varies from year to year, and students should check to see whether applying outside Ontario makes strategic sense for them.

I know an Ontario student who, after failing twice to get into medical school in his home province, moved to Alberta and established residency. Then, he applied and was accepted to one of the two medical schools in that province. He was determined to become a doctor in Canada and he found a way to make it happen.

Extreme? Perhaps. This kind of "loophole finding" is not uncommon among students applying today.

Students from other provinces or territories can apply to Ontario medical schools without restriction, since the majority of schools exist in Ontario. Many Ontario students don't like this rule, but that doesn't make it any less of a reality.

International students face even more barriers.

I met with a student recently who has been in Canada since age nine to go to school, billeting with Canadian families because her parents live in her home country. Now at university, she is paying international student fees in pursuit of a North American education that she can use in her home country or another country. She hopes this will include a medical education. Her parents don't want her to go to medical school in her home country because they feel it won't afford her the same opportunities.

However, only five medical schools accept international students to their programs (e.g., McGill, Memorial) and they tend to have single-digit numbers of spaces for them. This student is extremely limited in her options for where to apply (putting extreme pressure on her to be an extraordinary candidate), and, if she gets accepted, she will pay hefty international student fees. Further, if she's not established as a permanent resident in Canada by the time she applies for a medical residency, she may face challenges getting residency training: unlike domestic applicants, she may need a work permit.

Still, if I could choose a new doctor for myself, she might be it.

Hiring more doctors: a complicated equation

If there are too many applicants and not enough spaces, many students and parents wonder why "we" (government, universities, hospitals) don't just increase the medical-school class sizes so more applicants can get trained and more doctors can get hired to help fix the system.

As someone who was involved with recruiting physicians, I know that part of the answer to why it is so hard to get into medical school lies in what's at the end of medical school—and far beyond it.

For example, when I was recruiting physicians and we found someone we wanted to hire, I had to submit a Hospital Impact Analysis form. This was because every person we hired would be pressing on already constrained hospital resources, and we had to make sure that we could accommodate the new physician with the resources we had. This form included questions about operating room capacity, clinic space, equipment needs (e.g., Did we have enough MRI time to accommodate the new doctor's patients?), administrative and clerical support, lab space, personal office space, and much, much more.

In addition, medical schools need to ensure that they don't accept more medical students than the system across Canada can accommodate with residency spots. Residency is a necessary part of becoming a licensed physician and, even now, in some years, some medical students don't get a residency spot. That is a tragic situation for the affected students and, from my perspective, it's a good reason not to open up more medical-school spots.

Application evolution

Another factor that might make today's applicants less likely to succeed on their first try involves the evolution of the application process in Canada. I'll go into detail about the elements of applications, and strategies for them, in later chapters. Here, I want to talk generally about how things have changed.

"To be a good doctor, you just need to care about and be able to talk to people," a physician leader commented to me once. Possibly true—but it's understandably small comfort to students struggling to get their foot on the first rung of the process.

In years past, many applications to Canadian schools comprised some or all of the following elements: grade point average (GPA), Medical College Admission Test (MCAT) score, essays or short-answer questions, an autobiographical sketch (or CV or résumé), references, and interviews.

These elements also form part of applications today, but they have evolved in the twenty years I've been coaching medical-school hopefuls:

- A new MCAT came out in 2015, which includes topics that were not previously a focus (e.g., psychology, sociology).
- Only a few schools still ask for short-answer questions, a place where some students could shine.
- Some schools (e.g., McMaster, the University of Ottawa) use a web-based test: the Computer-based Assessment for Sampling Personal Characteristics (CASPer).
- Interviews usually have a "multiple mini" format now, versus the more common panel format of the past.

So, while the number of competitors might be similar to twenty years ago, the elements involved in the application process have a higher level of complexity, which can make standing out as a candidate very challenging now.

Underestimating the challenge

Many students I work with are incredibly hard working, do very well in school, and enter university on large scholarships. As high school students, they were among the top students in their region, if not the country. The same may be true of them once they enter university.

If they want into medical school, they have a lot of confidence that they will get into medical school: Why would they need help applying? *Of course*, they're going to be doctors! They are outstanding students, with scads of accolades.

I can't tell you how many parents have told me this at orientation events.

I can't tell you how many students have come to me during second-year university, when the realization hits that *a lot of other students are just like them* and that getting accepted to medical school will be tough.

They are the lucky ones—the ones who understand early in the game that this might not be the same as the other goals they have achieved.

I've worked with thousands of students who have come to me during their final year of university, trying to strategize around undergraduate grades that will not make the cut—even though their grades are relatively excellent. And it's hard to figure out how to fix things at that stage, because a GPA in medical school applications right now is almost always calculated from cumulative *undergraduate* grades.

That's right: most medical schools don't count graduate-school grades toward your GPA.

That's a lot of pressure on a student's undergraduate degree, at a time when a lot of other things are going on: finding your feet, growing up, adjusting to university workloads and evaluations, trying out different degree programs to see what fits, dealing with new illness or mental health issues, and living away from home the first time.

It is very common for students to have an adjustment period as they start university, but the current medical-school application process doesn't really allow for that normal life stage.

I believe these "I didn't get in—now what?" situations occur because most students (and parents) underestimate the challenge of applying to, interviewing for, and getting accepted to medical school—*especially the first time*. Further, it can bear little resemblance to the level of competition or difficulty that their physician friends or family members went through even twenty years ago.

For many of these reasons, many "successful" students don't get in, especially on their first attempt.

The repercussions from that include loss of application money, effort, and preparation time, and having to wait an entire year to apply again—and, perhaps most crucially, loss of confidence.

> **INSIDER INSIGHT**
>
> It's not a failure to get rejected from medical school the first time. It's **the norm**.

Notes

1. "Medical School Application Statistics," Ontario Universities' Application Centre, updated November 13, 2017, https://www.ouac.on.ca/statistics/med_app_stats/.

2. Association of Faculties of Medicine of Canada, *Canadian Medical Education Statistics* (Ottawa: Association of Faculties of Medicine of Canada, 2017 [vol. 39]), 101.

3

Why do you want to be a doctor?

You think you'll apply to medical school, or you are applying or have applied. But have you really thought about the big question: **Why do you want to be a doctor?**

Such a simple question—such a difficult question to answer. Usually, when I have asked students this question, whether in an advising situation or a medical-school interview, they stumble.

"Um...I like science?"

"Uh...I want to help people?"

"Like...(gulp)...someone told me I'd make a good one?"

"And...my mom is one. What she does looks...um...cool?"

"Also...I want a job where I can keep learning."

I interviewed medical-school candidates as part of a panel that included, at times, a (somewhat grumpy) physician. When he heard answers like this, let me tell you what he did: he just grunted.

If you're still in high school, the big question can be particularly challenging. You're still trying to get through that English class your guidance counsellor told you to take! But, the reality is that answering this question may not get any easier when you're an undergraduate or in graduate school.

Lots of amazing people, similar to you, want to become physicians. This doesn't diminish anything about you, but it can make it challenging to come across as a memorable and unique candidate. Taking time to really investigate this career, and solidify why it is a great fit for you, is time well spent—for your mental health, as well as for your applications and interviews.

Why get clarity?

During my time screening candidates for medical-school admission, I considered asking why a candidate wanted to be a doctor a standard question. These days, you may never hear or see this question during your application and interview process—at least, not directly. That doesn't mean you don't need good clarity around your answer.

Why is it important to think about the reasons you want to be a doctor? Why is it important to have an articulate answer? Here are just a few reasons:

- **Applying to medical school is extremely competitive in Canada.** It's a fairly lengthy, stressful, expensive, and time-consuming process. Knowing the answer to why you want to be a doctor can help you on those days when you wonder, "Why am I doing this, again?" If you have the answer to the big question, it will help you refocus and reenergize.
- **When you apply, you will be asked to submit information about yourself.** You will need to describe and reflect on your activities and experiences. Whether it's in the application process or interviews, knowing the answer to why you want to be a doctor can really help you and others understand the rationale and motivation behind your experiences. I believe this tends to lead to better scoring and better chances of getting accepted.
- **Knowing the answer is a checkmark on the "informed candidate" list.** That's a good thing. Every year, I have worked with at least one upper-year medical student who comes to see me because they have realized that they don't want to be a doctor. They are usually sweaty and terrified and in great distress. Can you imagine? All that work and effort to get in, all the learning and money to go through medical school, all the hopes and dreams (yours and others')—all for nothing.

Leaving medical school or deciding not to work as a physician is an extremely stressful, major life decision. I don't wish it on anyone. It's also a huge waste of money—your money, your medical school's money, and government and taxpayer's money. We've partially trained you and now we're going to lose all that investment.

While there aren't massive numbers of students in this situation, there are some. When I screened candidates for medical-school admissions, I thought about these students. I looked at candidates and wondered, Do they really know why they want to do this? Are they truly informed about what's facing them? In other words, I wanted to know (and I'm sure everyone who does medical-school admissions still wants to know), Will they be happy in this program and career? Will they go all the way?

The common answers to the big question: not enough

Let's get you thinking about this for a moment, by brainstorming the reasons you want to become a physician (see the exercise that follows).

EXERCISE: WHY DO YOU WANT TO BE A DOCTOR? (PART 1)

Let's ignore the grumpy physician I described earlier. I'd like you to simply brainstorm answers to why you want to be a doctor. Don't worry about whether they are the "right" answers or whether they would pass a medical-school admissions review. Just get as many answers down as you can.

If you come up with lots of ideas in the brainstorming exercise, great. If you have trouble writing anything down, take heart: this chapter aims to help you start figuring things out.

If you were able to write something down, ask yourself a new question: Could anyone else applying to medical school have the same answers as me?

Based on my experience, yes. That's not catastrophic, and I'm going to help you, but here's why it's a problem for your answers to resemble those of other candidates. People involved with medical-school admissions review many applications (at certain points, potentially thousands) and interview many candidates. I'm sure it makes sense that the candidates have similarities. They've all taken on the same ambitious goal of getting into medical school, after all, and there are specific requirements to apply. It's reasonable that people with similar interests would find a career as a physician motivating. On top of that, and related to it, most of you are from similar academic programs (something in the sciences) and have very similar extracurricular activities—again, partly because you're attracted to many of the same kinds of things.

When the people involved with medical-school admissions go to review your application or interview you, it can incredibly difficult for you to stand out. You're part of a talented pool of students, and most of you look very similar on paper and, sometimes, in person.

It's also understandable that someone who thinks about a career as a physician likes science, wants to help people, has been influenced by other people's interesting-looking careers, wants to continually learn, and so on.

So, how do you make your answer authentic and stand out?

Here's what I believe: you have to **connect your (very common) answers to your own experiences** and what you have learned from them. That is the part that is unique to you.

I'll describe more about how to harness your unique experiences later in this chapter and in other chapters.

If the brainstorming exercise was a blank for you, you probably need to explore the physician-as-career option more before you apply. You don't want the admissions people to write down, "Great student, not ready yet."

Getting beyond the common answers

Testing your fit with the role of physician

I remember working with a student years ago who had just completed a four-year degree in physical therapy. She came to see me because she was not happy in that field.

"I've realized that I don't like touching people," she confessed to me, as we started to work on some other career ideas for her. When I asked her if she had considered any other options yet, she said, "Well, I was thinking of becoming a doctor."

This is an example of what happens when people don't explore down to the details and tasks of a job idea.

It can be challenging to know what goes on inside a job day to day, but there are ways you can *start* to test out the role of physician.

- **Consider volunteering in health-care or hospital settings** to assess your level of comfort with those environments and observe more about what people do (physicians and others).
- **Consider working or volunteering in patient-centred environments.** For example, many students work or volunteer in nursing homes, with people with disabilities, with children, with vulnerable people (e.g., refugees, prison inmates, sexual assault survivors, campus detox rooms, campus medical outreach services, campus sexual health services, and so on).

These are great ways to establish relationships and gain experience. Perhaps even more importantly, they let you test your reaction to body fluids, illness, odours, and touching people. Even if you end up in a relatively office-based medical specialty, you still have to get through medical school and residency, where your training will involve body fluids and all the rest.

WAYS TO TEST THE FIT AND SOUND INFORMED

Beware the trap of "hospital experience," however. I believe that working in community health-care or hospital environments is excellent experience for potential medical students, but I know that physicians sometimes challenge the value of that experience.

One student reported to me, after a medical-school interview, that she explained her goal of becoming a doctor partly by describing her experience as a hospital volunteer. A physician on the interview panel responded that his job wasn't about "bringing people juice" and questioned how she knew that *physician* was the job for her.

> **INSIDER INSIGHT**
> Hospital experience is valuable. But, on its own, it may not demonstrate that you really understand why this particular role is right for you.

Here are some other ways you can gain more information about what physicians do:

- **Talk to family members or friends who are physicians.** Ask them about their daily tasks, what they find most exciting, most difficult, most frustrating.
- **Request meetings with medical students, residents, or physicians** to ask them about their work (many people make an appointment with their family doctor, to start).

- **Pursue opportunities for observerships or job shadowing.**
  This is where you ask to follow someone around for a period,
  to see what their work looks like. Because there are confiden-
  tiality and privacy issues involved in providing medical care,
  you could approach teaching hospitals (hospitals affiliated
  with medical schools): they are more likely to have processes
  in place that allow job shadowing.

Step 1 in answering the question of why you want to be a doctor is
to understand and articulate more about what is specific to the role
of doctor. Use research from books, websites, and meetings with
people to build a good picture of what physicians do that is unique
to their role. Write a list that answers the question: What do physicians do that other health-care providers don't do?

Step 2 is to reflect on what you have seen and heard. How does
it connect with what you know about yourself? For example, you
could set up a table like this:

WHAT I LEARNED FROM THE DOCTORS I OBSERVED/TALKED TO	WHEN HAVE I EXPERIENCED THIS IN MY OWN LIFE?
Need to be good at talking to and connecting with people (family doc)	When I volunteered with the suicide hot-line, I had to connect to people quickly and sensitively.

Exploring other heath-care careers

Many times, the answers students give for why they want to be a doctor fit many roles other than doctor. For example, you may answer
that you love science and helping people. Why not consider being a
nurse, a physical therapist, a dentist, an optometrist, a pharmacist,
an X-ray technologist, a hospital administrator, or a perfusionist?

Many medical-school applicants have told me, "I want a
job where I can be challenged
and learn all the time." I have
responded that they should
consider career counselling,
because I feel that those are
integral parts of my job!

INSIDER INSIGHT

It's important to explore other
career options, so you can
effectively answer why *physician* is
the best role for you and to show
that you have eliminated other
options in an informed way.

Exploring other careers can be helpful for other reasons, too. As you know, most students apply more than once before they are accepted to medical school. Career options give you something to pursue while you're waiting to reapply, and an alternate plan if, ultimately, you never get accepted. In fact, these options can lead to satisfying careers.

I worked with a student who didn't get into medical school the first time he applied. After analyzing his application, he decided it was mostly because his grade point average wasn't competitive. Since medical schools currently emphasize undergraduate grades, we talked about options for more undergraduate courses. He was really interested in the patient-care part of being a physician—helping people in distress, helping to prevent illness and disease, caring for people. Since he was graduating from a science program, I asked him if he had ever considered doing a fast-track nursing degree.

He was taken aback, as many students thinking of medical school are. Wasn't that just "settling" for something inferior? Every time I mention nursing to medical-school hopefuls, I see a look that I call "Smart people don't become nurses, do they?" This student and I talked about the fact that a nursing degree would enable him to work directly with patients in clinical settings, giving him many of the job elements he was seeking through medical school. It would also allow him to gain clinical experience and credibility (and money!) while he reapplied to medical school in the future.

He was excited and got accepted into a nursing program. He later confessed to me that he had taken this path only as a "GPA enhancer" until he could reapply to medical school. It was a means to an end. But something happened while he was being educated to be a nurse. He realized that it was, in fact, the role he had wanted all along. He was exposed to the differences—not better or worse—between what physicians and nurses do, and he realized that he wanted to do nursing. He now works as a nurse and has not reapplied to medical school.

Yes, indeed, smart people do become nurses, and have fulfilling and respected careers.

I tell you this story, not to discourage you from becoming a physician, but because

ASK YOURSELF
What are my biases about other health-care careers? Have I learned about other options? Have I dismissed other options prematurely?

many smart students float or are pushed toward becoming physicians as if it's the only direction they can go. They're not aware of the many other interesting, fulfilling, and lucrative health-related jobs that exist.

RESOURCES FOR EXPLORING OTHER HEALTH-CARE CAREERS

Here are a few resources to help you investigate the hundreds of other health-related careers that also might be a good fit for you.

WEBSITES

Healthecareers.com: This website is a job board for people working in health care. It's a great way to get a sense of the many clinical and nonclinical roles involved in working in hospitals and health environments.

Charityvillage.com: Want to help people? This website has jobs for people working in community-based settings, often with a health focus, although it also covers broader social justice, humanitarian, and international types of work.

CareerCruising.com: Ask if your high school or university has a subscription to this site. You can explore the roles it lists in the "health" section, and it has basic job descriptions, educational requirements, video interviews with people who do the work, salary information, and more.

BOOKS

Here is a selection of books that might help (this is by no means comprehensive). Some of them have been around a while—the *Careers for* series, for example. I recommend you give them a try all the same. They are very accessible—and their starting points (noting things that characterize you) may be your starting points.

> *Top 100 Health-Careers* by Saul Wischnitzer and Edith Wischnitzer (Jist Publishing, 2005)
>
> *Careers for Scientific Types and Others with Inquiring Minds* by Jan Goldberg (McGraw-Hill Education, 2007)
>
> *Careers for Caring People and Other Sensitive Types* by Adrian Paradis (McGraw-Hill Education, 2003)
>
> *Hot Healthcare Careers: 30 Occupations with Fast Growth and Many New Job Openings* by Andrew Morkes (College and Career Press, 2017)
>
> *101 Careers in Healthcare Management* by Leonard Friedman and Anthony R. Kovner (Springer, 2012)

Career options outside health care

Some students who aim for medical school have no interest in health care if they can't become physicians. I have to confess that, thinking as a patient, these students make me nervous: If their next-choice careers have nothing to do with health care, do I want them as my future doctor?

My own opinions aside, if you are one of the people who loves the puzzles of medicine, and the prestige, the salary, and the challenge, I urge you to investigate more about whether the reality lives up to the hype. Maybe it does. Maybe it's not quite what you thought.

Then, remember there are other careers that involve these elements, too. I have spoken with students applying to medical school who, if they didn't get in, wanted to do a master's of business administrative (MBA). It was the "running a business" part of the role that appealed to them. Engineers apply to medical school and, if unsuccessful, often continue in their technical field—sometimes with a health element (e.g., prosthetics, ergonomics, medical product design) and sometimes without. Political science students may go on to do a health policy degree or work in patient advocacy. Psychology students often work in other clinical settings (e.g., clinical psychology, counselling psychology, medical social work) or community-based settings (e.g., community support worker, patient liaison, education coordinator, program manager).

Career options come from exploring what's "out there," as well as understanding more about yourself and what you are really looking for. Check with your school guidance office or campus career centre for more help.

Why not one of those options, instead?

Now that you have some sense of other career possibilities, you can start to effectively answer when people ask you, "Well, why not do one of those things, instead of being a doctor?"

I'm not trying to discourage you from these other career options. One or more of them might be really great for you. If you still want to be a doctor, though, you need to know what those options lack from your point of view—and, therefore, why *physician* is best for you. Thinking this through can also help you make better decisions about your future and come across as a more informed, lower-risk candidate to medical-school admissions personnel. I encourage you to think it through in writing. Here's another table you could set up:

WHAT I LEARNED FROM THE DOCTORS I OBSERVED/TALKED TO	WHEN HAVE I EXPERIENCED THIS IN MY OWN LIFE?	WHAT OTHER WORK ROLES WOULD VALUE THIS SKILL?	WHY ARE THEY NOT THE RIGHT FIT FOR ME?
Need to be good at talking to and connecting with people (family doc)	When I volunteered with the suicide hotline, I had to connect to people quickly and sensitively.	Nursing Social worker	Nursing: not enough diagnostic tasks Social worker: too much referring, not enough fixing

I also encourage you to revisit the brainstorming exercise on why you want to be a doctor (see the exercise that follows).

EXERCISE: WHY DO YOU WANT TO BE A DOCTOR? (PART 2)

This is still not an easy question to answer, but I hope you have gained some insights into what makes it an effective and helpful answer—for you and for an application committee.

Your answer needs to take into consideration:

- why **not** something else that's similar
- why **doctor** is the specific role that is the best fit
- how your answer will sound unique, relative to other candidates (hint: it's **your** experiences that are unique)
- specific examples from your life that show the fit with being a doctor

Brainstorm ideas under the following topics to help you formulate your answer:

Tasks I like doing that (only) physicians get to do

How I found out what doctors do (experiences I've gathered and resources I've used)

My personality fit with what physicians get to do

What others say I'm good at

My specific examples: proof from my life experiences of my fit with what physicians get to do

My future life goals that match what physicians get to do

4

The application process in Canada

Application timelines

In Canada, you need to complete some or all of an undergraduate (bachelor's) degree before you can apply to medical school. Many students ask me: When is the best year to apply?

That depends. Bear in mind that you will need to meet the minimum entrance requirements for the schools to which you want to apply. For example, the current norm at Memorial University is a complete undergraduate degree at the time of admission. The University of British Columbia recommends at least ninety undergraduate credits—often equivalent to three full-time years of study.

You can apply in advance, as long as you will have completed the requirements for admission by the time of admission. So, if you are hoping to enter medical school after your final year of a four-year degree, you apply **during** your final year of that degree.

Despite meeting the minimum academic entrance requirements, you will also need to assess when the best year is for **you** to apply. This will be based on the details of your particular situation (I discuss this more in later chapters).

In Ontario, the medical-school application process is centralized through the Ontario Medical School Application Service (OMSAS), a part of the Ontario Universities' Application Centre (OUAC) website. At the moment, the deadline for application to OMSAS (and any Ontario medical school) is October 1 of the year before you anticipate starting medical school.

Outside Ontario, candidates apply to each school separately and the deadlines vary.

Typical timelines by type of candidate

UNDERGRADUATE STUDENTS (MOST OF YOU)

Most students enter medical school after completing some or all of an undergraduate degree. This is because most Canadian medical schools now require a four-year degree before candidates qualify for admission.[1] Many students apply during their final year of a four-year degree. Lots of students apply in the year following graduation from their undergraduate degree (or later). Some apply during their third year of an undergraduate degree (depending on the school and if they qualify).

GRADUATE STUDENTS (MANY OF YOU)

There are many students enrolled in graduate programs (master's, professional, and PhD) who want to apply to medical school. Most medical schools have supplementary documentation or processes for these applicants. You may have to submit a letter from your graduate supervisor indicating that they are aware of and support your application to medical school. You may have to submit a curriculum vitae and information about your graduate work. Although there are always exceptions to every rule, medical schools will not allow you to leave your graduate program to attend medical school. I think they want to prevent students from using graduate programs as stepping-stones to get into medical school—programs they abandon (unfairly and at significant cost to the programs) once admitted to medical school. Some students do apply during their graduate work, but they defer entrance to medical school until completion of their graduate degree.

HIGH SCHOOL STUDENTS APPLYING TO QUEEN'S UNIVERSITY ACCELERATED ROUTE TO MEDICAL SCHOOL (A HIGHLY SELECT GROUP OF YOU)

One of my medical colleagues once commented that he sometimes worried about the reproductive health of medical students and residents, since gaining admission to medical school tends to take so long and often pushes having children to a later age. He might have been relieved, therefore, to hear about the Queen's University Accelerated Route to Medical School (QuARMS)—a program that shortens the journey to full licensing. Up to ten spots are allocated for this program. Students apply in high school and meet a rigorous set of criteria for admission. When they graduate high school, they complete two years of an undergraduate degree in arts, sciences, or computing at Queen's University, and then start medical school at Queen's. Visit the QuARMS website for more information (use *QuARMS* as the search term in your browser).

MATURE STUDENTS (VERY FEW OF YOU)

I have met a few students in this category in my advising practice. One student, in particular, comes to mind. He immigrated to Canada in his forties as a tradesperson. In Canada, he went back to school and completed a high school diploma, an undergraduate degree, and medical school. I met him when he was applying for residency. He wanted to be a family doctor and he succeeded—at a time of life when many people would have assumed that a career change, especially to a career with lengthy training, was impossible.

My former family doctor was a teacher before she was a doctor. I've also worked with quite a few PhD graduates (one with a PhD in biochemistry jumps to mind) who, after years in their original field, went to medical school. Everyone's path is different. "Mature" students still need to meet medical-school requirements, of course. If you are in this category, I encourage you to pursue your path: becoming a physician is an achievable goal. Some applicants return to undergraduate work to take science courses, as in the case of a PhD English graduate I worked with—she wanted to qualify as a candidate at more medical schools. I think this may have also showed the medical schools just how committed this student was to her new path.

Many undergraduate students are in a huge rush to get into medical school and, while I understand many of the reasons for this, I encourage everyone to consider that medical school might remain an achievable dream long after the typical applicant is admitted.

Application elements

Every school uses some or all of the following elements to assess candidates. However, which they use and how they use them varies by school and by year. Be sure to check the websites of each medical school that interests you to find out what they will be assessing during the year you plan to apply.

Grade point average and prerequisite courses

Every medical school assesses your GPA, but not every school has a minimum requirement (or will divulge it). I suspect this is because the applicant pool varies from year to year, and there are always exceptions to the general "excellent candidate" profile. Schools need the flexibility to respond to these exceptions. This lack of clarity around GPA, however, makes things murky for candidates trying to figure out if they qualify on a school's GPA scale.

Generally:

- GPA almost solely considers undergraduate grades (but the University of Toronto is an example of a school that gives a small amount of credit to graduate grades).

- GPA is usually cumulative and often includes grades from the first year of university, which is a transition year for many people (but Queen's University is an example of a school that currently reviews grades from only the final two years of university, if you don't meet the minimum cumulative cutoff).

- You will likely need to "convert" your university's method of grading to a scale preferred by the medical school. This is centralized in Ontario, and individualized by school in other provinces. This can make it challenging to figure out how "qualified" your GPA is, because these conversion scales are not very precise.

As you can probably tell, there are many exceptions to these general guidelines. Each candidate has to do homework to figure out how their GPA measures up at medical schools, which is part of figuring out where they have the best chance for admission.

Some schools also have prerequisite courses: you have to do these courses before they will consider you. Often, these courses (such as biology, chemistry, and organic chemistry) are included in a basic science curriculum, but you should check the prerequisite courses specified by each school to which you want to apply. For one thing, you don't have to major in the sciences to apply to medical school. For another, some schools may require an English course, a humanities course, or something that you might not expect. You can take prerequisites in any year of your program, as long as they are at the level that the medical school stipulates (e.g., a required first-year biology course could be taken during your third year, if that's when it fits your schedule).

Medical College Admissions Test

Most schools in Canada require some or all of the MCAT as part of their application process. This test was revised in 2015 and many schools only accept the 2015 version, while others still allow the former version—at least, for now.

The MCAT is run through a US-based organization called the Association of American Medical Colleges. The test has several sections. Some schools assess each section's scores, as well as the total score, as part of your application (e.g., Dalhousie University currently does this). Other schools review only one section of the test (e.g., the University of Calgary currently assesses only the section on critical analysis and reasoning).

Many candidates write the MCAT more than once. Schools have different approaches to repeated MCATs. Some schools calculate a cumulative score from all your MCATs to arrive at a total score (e.g., the University of Alberta currently does this), while others only take your most recent score.

Your MCAT scores remain valid for a finite amount of time, so check with each school about whether a past MCAT score (or indeed, the pre-2015 version of the MCAT) will count in their application process.

Autobiographical sketch, curriculum vitae, or résumé

As part of the application process, you usually have to provide information that helps the admissions committee assess your personal qualities and characteristics. This is often done by requesting an autobiographical sketch, or sometimes a CV or résumé. In Ontario, all schools currently require at least a basic autobiographical sketch, and some also request and review additional details about items in your sketch.

In Ontario, the format of the sketch typically asks candidates to list activities from age sixteen onwards. Some medical schools are also interested in more detailed reflection on some of these activities (e.g., the University of Toronto has recently been requesting candidates to submit three brief statements on the activities from their sketch that best exemplify attributes that align with four specific "clusters").

Since the autobiographical sketch starts at age sixteen, most candidates have to include activities from their time in high school—a time when the specifics of a medical-school application weren't yet top of mind. This can lead to complications when the candidates are asked to submit the next element of the sketch, CV, or résumé: verifiers.

VERIFIERS

Verifiers are people who can verify your involvement in the activities you list in your sketch, CV, or résumé. OMSAS—the centralized Ontario Medical School Application Service— asks you to submit names and contact information for verifiers. Many schools require verifiers for at least some activities in your sketch, CV, or résumé. Other schools require verifiers for **every** activity. This can pose problems: maybe the teacher who coached your volleyball team has left their position, or the neighbour you babysat for in high school doesn't live next door anymore. To find verifiers, you may have to chase a lot of people down, and it can get time-consuming and stressful to take care of these details in your applications.

> **TIPS FOR HIGH SCHOOL AND EARLY UNIVERSITY**
>
> Starting to think about your autobiographical sketch in high school and early university can help you remember to stay in touch with people, so you can use them as verifiers later on.

Computer-based Assessment for Sampling Personal Characteristics

A few medical schools are now using an online assessment, the Computer-based Assessment for Sampling Personal Characteristics (CASPer), as part of their application process (e.g., McMaster University, the University of Ottawa, and Dalhousie University). I think the use of CASPer might increase in the future, as medical schools grapple with lots of candidates and continue to refine their assessment processes.

At medical schools that use it, CASPer is a stage of the application process that happens before the interview stage. Students log in at a specified date and time, and provide timed, typed responses to video-based and written scenarios.

McMaster University has quite extensive help for students

preparing for CASPer on their website, so visit the website to get a sense of what this process looks like.

References

Medical schools are interested in students who can work with other people. Perhaps this is why references are a part of the application process. In Ontario, where the process is centralized, each of your referees is asked to complete a confidential assessment form. Referees submit the forms to OMSAS, which then forwards these with the rest of your application to each medical school to which you have applied.

I encourage students to think of letters of reference as *letters of recommendation*. If you have a choice about whom to pick as a referee, choose people who will not merely write about you, but will recommend you wholeheartedly and enthusiastically.

Medical schools often ask for three references, so think about cultivating and maintaining those relationships early.

Special-category documents

To strive for a physician workforce in Canada that represents the population it serves, medical schools identify special categories for some admissions. The type and number of special-category admissions vary from school to school. Special-category candidates must meet the basic criteria of the schools to which they apply. They then undergo additional assessment. Schools may require them to submit additional documentation. Examples of special categories include:

- applicants of African descent (some medical schools call this category "Black applicants")
- Indigenous applicants
- graduate-student applicants
- applicants to combined programs (e.g., MD/PhD, MD/JD, MD/MPA, and more)
- international applicants
- military applicants (not applicable every application cycle)

If you identify with a category on this list (or more than one category), you may wish to consult the specific requirements for applying under that category. You will still need to meet the rigorous merit criteria of the medical schools to which you apply, of course.

Interviews

All Canadian medical schools count interviews as part of their assessment process. Despite their high cost in time and money, interviews help identify factors in applicants that can't be assessed through other application elements.

For medical schools in Canada, interviewing mostly happens between January and April. However, some schools may interview you over the December holiday break, assuming you are close to your home province at that time (e.g., Dalhousie University seems to have done this in the past).

At the moment, there seem to be three main types of interview formats:

- **Multiple mini-interviews (MMIs)** represent the most common interview format. They form all or part of the interview process at many schools. MMIs sort of simulate a medical clinic, with multiple rooms or stations (often eight to thirteen) where you meet people and answer questions or deal with a scenario.

   In many MMIs, you have two minutes to read a prompt outside a room, and then eight minutes to enter the room and respond to the question or scenario. At the end of the eight minutes, you move to the next room and begin the process again. After you have completed half the mini-interviews, you often get a break.

   McMaster University pioneered MMIs in 2002, and MMIs have since been adopted across Canada, in the United States, and internationally. Research at McMaster has subsequently shown that this type of interviewing increases the overall reliability in judging a candidate's merits, and reduces the effect of a "mistake" an applicant might show in a single interaction.[2]

- **Panel interviews** are what medical-school interviewing used to most commonly involve. The panels I volunteered with included a faculty member (often an MD or PhD from the sciences), a second- or third-year medical student, and a community member (that was my role). Some schools that have used panel interviews have a two-person panel, omitting the community member (e.g., Western University has recently used this format).

- **Combined-format interviews** may involve MMIs plus a panel interview. Queen's University did this in the past: candidates went through a somewhat-shortened MMI sequence and a short panel interview. Other combined formats may involve MMIs or a panel interview plus a written response to a question.

Application outcomes

There is probably little that is more anticipated by medical-school applicants than the holy grail of an acceptance letter.

This usually happens in May. However, as with everything, it varies by school. This means any backup plans you have on the horizon (e.g., going to graduate school, working, travelling) may have to remain uncertain until after you know the status of your application to medical school.

Acceptance can take a few forms. Because you have likely applied to more than one school, and many other applicants have as well, you and other candidates might receive more than one offer. The offers you reject go back into the system, so that other qualified students can be offered your rejected spots.

Waiting lists

Because of the likelihood that some candidates will receive more than one offer, you may be wait-listed. This means that a medical school has ranked you among their accepted candidates, but you didn't score high enough to be among their first wave of offers.

Candidates sometimes hear very late in the game that they have been ultimately accepted or rejected. Some medical schools give you a sense of the timelines involved in their particular process—such as your position in the waiting-list queue—so you can get a handle on your next steps.

Rejection

Unfortunately, the statistics tell us that the odds are against you getting accepted the first time you apply to medical school. However, there is considerable information you can glean from the rejection process that can help you when and if you reapply. Rest assured that most candidates apply twice and some even more. It is a very normal part of this process—don't interpret rejection to your first round of applications as failure.

If you applied to a reasonable number of schools and didn't get offered any interviews, this normally points to one of the following problems:

- You didn't apply to enough schools, or you didn't apply to the right schools (i.e., schools where you actually met the criteria).
- Your GPA and/or MCAT score were not competitive enough for this year's applicant pool.
- Your additional application elements were not competitive enough for this year's applicant pool.

ASK YOURSELF

Is there anything I can improve or change for the next round?

Will there be a next round for me?

Where can I seek help?

If you got one or more interviews and you didn't get accepted, take heart. While disappointing to be sure, it is generally a good sign that you got to the interview stage. You may need to work on your interview strategies and presentation before you apply again. When I screened applicants for medical-school admission, the number of applicants in the interview stage was double or triple the number the school could actually accept.

Most medical schools won't give you detailed feedback (if any) on a rejected application, but a few will give you some sense of where your application didn't meet the applicant-pool standard that year.

Acceptance

If you are lucky enough to be offered spots at multiple schools, you will need to decide which one to accept. Once you accept, it is theoretically possible, but very difficult, to transfer to another school later. Because medical school is so competitive to get into, many candidates don't give much thought to the reasons for applying to a particular place. For many, it's more a case of "I met the minimum criteria there" and not about the location or program itself.

This is a time, if you haven't already researched it, to figure out whether this location and program is for you. Each medical school has a certain culture. They are all slightly different sizes. What will work best for you?

ASK YOURSELF

Do I prefer smaller class sizes or bigger class sizes?

Think about the social events that went with interviews. What did they help me learn about the school, the people, and the location?

Do I prefer to be in a large urban centre?

How will living close to home or far away affect the way I manage the stress, and the academic and financial demands, of medical school?

Do the students in the program I'm considering have good residency match rates? (Do they mostly get in to what they want, where they want? Do many go unmatched?) Check the CaRMS website for information about each medical school's match rates.

DEFERRING

Most medical schools will not let you defer your admission, unless you have a very serious and compelling reason. The most common reason for deferral (though not always granted) is that you are finishing a graduate program. The only way to know if a school might consider this is to check with the school (I recommend doing this by reading their website to see what they say about deferral, or calling them by phone so that you are somewhat anonymous). More importantly, I would check with the school *before* you apply, not when you get the acceptance offer.

You will not likely get a deferral to finish an undergraduate program, or to travel, work, or do something else. There are too many other applicants eager to accept immediately.

Notes

1. Association of Faculties of Medicine of Canada. *Admission Requirements of Canadian Faculties of Medicine 2018*. Ottawa, ON, Canada.
2. "Multiple Mini-Interview (MMI)," McMaster University, accessed June 2, 2018, https://mdprogram.mcmaster.ca/md-program-admissions/how-we-select/multiple-mini-interview-(mmi).

5

Finances

If I asked you how you intend to pay for medical school, what would you say?

This question might seem like an invasion of privacy, but I have heard it asked during a medical-school interview. It's not really a question about your bank account, but rather a question about whether you have thought past the "getting in" part of this process. Have you started to plan for success by working out how you will cover the costs of this extravaganza called medical school? Do you know that medical-school tuition in Canada has been deregulated? Deregulation means that some professional programs at some universities—including law, engineering, and medicine—have higher tuition than other university programs. It allows universities to charge close to the true costs of these professional programs, because students graduating from these programs are generally compensated by employment with higher pay.

But first you have to get to the part where you pay tuition! Simply applying for medical school has costs. It's worth factoring these costs into your plans. This chapter will help you approximate what you need to budget for. The costs described here are not guaranteed to be accurate, especially over the long term, so you need to check with each institution to get the most current information.

If cost is preventing you from applying to, or attending, medical school, some subsidies (not many) are available. This chapter covers those as well.

Application-process costs

Costs related to the Medical College Admission Test

STUDY COSTS

Preparing for the MCAT can cost anywhere from $200 to $11,000.

Most students prepare for the MCAT through self-study (i.e., by buying or borrowing books) or by taking a prep course (in person or online). If you borrow books from a library or a friend, be sure to note the date of the publication: you need something that teaches the 2015 version of the MCAT, and the more recent the publication, the better.

If you choose to buy books or take a course, this costs money. For example, I found MCAT prep courses for $595 (22 hours), $845 (40 hours), and more ($1,799, $2,299). Some estimates report that prep courses can cost up to $11,000, depending on extras you sign up for, such as private tutoring and additional help on certain sections. Some companies that market courses offer guarantees—for example, if you don't get the grades you need, the next course is free, or reduced in price, or they will give you your money back.

Books currently seem to range from $177 to $800, so they are generally a cheaper option than courses. Most books have some sort of online component. I've had many students remark that buying and borrowing books from a range of MCAT-prep providers helped them study in a more comprehensive way, because different resources emphasized different topics. This could increase costs, if you are buying.

Use due diligence: read reviews, and ask friends about their experiences with courses and books, before you hand over your money.

TAKING THE SUMMER OFF OR REDUCING WORK TO STUDY

In addition to the cost of study supplies, you need to consider the cost of taking time off to study. Many students report taking off an entire summer to study for their exam. This means loss of a summer's earnings, which is not insignificant. A student who works a 35-hour week during the 16-week break from university—even at minimum wage—faces more than $7,500 in lost income. Of course, you may not have the luxury of taking the summer off to study, but any reduction in time working will have a financial impact. It makes sense to figure out what that impact will be, so you are prepared.

EXAMINATION COSTS

In 2018, the MCAT cost $315 USD, if you registered far enough in advance. The cost increased to $370 USD, if you left it until eight days before the exam. Other potential costs include cancellation fees, fees for changing test dates, and international-student fees (international-student fees don't apply to Canadian students).

Application fees

Let's talk about application fees in Ontario first. This makes sense because all students across Canada are eligible for spots in Ontario medical schools. In other provinces, almost all spots are reserved for residents of those provinces.

The Ontario application process is centralized through OMSAS. There is currently a base fee of $220 CAD plus additional fees for each university in Ontario to which you apply (between $100 and $125 each). If you apply to all six Ontario medical schools, your total application fee is $920 plus transcript fees.

Outside Ontario, you pay a processing fee to each medical school you apply to (e.g., $70 for Dalhousie University, $90 for the University of Saskatchewan, $150 for the University of Calgary).

Transcripts

For applications to Ontario medical schools, OMSAS currently charges $12 per transcript request. You are required to request transcripts from any postsecondary institution you have attended. For many students, this fee totals only $12—but if you attended more than one university, factor that cost into your total.

Medical schools outside Ontario also charge for transcripts. Check with each medical school for their rates.

No matter where you apply, foreign transcripts (outside Canada) may involve additional fees.

Volunteering costs and lost work

A large part of any medical-school application is information about your experience and activities. Volunteering in your community can be an important part of building this element of your application. Later chapters cover ways you can get involved in your community that aren't necessarily formally structured volunteer "jobs"— and needn't cost you in lost wages. However, typical volunteering (e.g., two hours every week at a retirement home) can be at the expense of paid work (perhaps up to $2,000), so give this some attention because it can sneak up on you.

Travel costs for interviews

If you are lucky enough to be invited for interviews, you may have travel costs, especially if you are interviewing at more than one school. Schools often interview in the same brief time period, which can make airline and train tickets more expensive than if you could space out your trips. Travel might cost you upwards of $3,000. On top of getting to your destination, you may be paying for hotels, meals, and taxis or transit fare.

Clothing for interviews

Most students wear clothing to their interviews that is not their typical daily outfit. It's important to present the best version of yourself—competent, tidy, and professional. You may be buying shoes, and a suit or dress. You may need tailoring, or dry cleaning, or a haircut. This might add up to $1,000 or more. If you are borrowing clothes, be sure to wear them around your house first to check for comfort, fit, and cleanliness, so that you feel your best on interview day.

EXERCISE: BUDGETING FOR APPLICATION-PROCESS COSTS

Build a budget chart for application-process costs.

In a column, make a list of the following items:

Study costs: prep courses, books

Taking time off, or reducing work, to study

Application fees (list fees for each school you want to apply to)

Transcripts

Volunteering costs

Interview travel costs: travel tickets, accommodation, food, and taxi or transit fare

Interview clothing: purchased outfit, purchased shoes, haircut or style, dry cleaning, tailoring

Other

After each item, describe its potential cost, your budget for it, and the date when you need to pay for it.

Application and interview scholarships

It's worth checking for scholarships and bursaries to help you with the costs of the MCAT, and applications and interviews, if these costs are prohibitive for you.

- The Association of Faculties of Medicine of Canada (AFMC) offers approximately 700 awards to Canadian students in financial need to reduce the cost of writing the MCAT. (For more information, use the search term *AFMC MCAT assistance* in your browser.)

- The Association of American Medical Colleges (AAMC) Fee Assistance Program offers help with MCAT and other fees, if you are applying to schools through the American Medical College Application Service (AMCAS-US). You are eligible for this assistance if you are a US citizen (dual citizens are considered US citizens). (For more information, use the search term *AAMC fee assistance* in your browser.)

> **INSIDER INSIGHT**
> Contact student awards at the universities to which you are applying—and the medical schools themselves—for other sources of funding to help with the cost of applications and interviews for students in need. Some sort of assistance is definitely possible. Medical schools do not want financial constraints to disadvantage or prevent students from applying or interviewing.

Approximate cost of medical school

I have heard, anecdotally, that many Ontario (and other) students start medical school with zero debt, and graduate with $100,000 of debt. If you weren't fortunate enough to graduate with zero debt after your first degree, this figure can be even higher. Why so expensive? Medical-school tuition has been deregulated in some provinces (a process that results in some programs, like medicine, not being subject to the same tuition caps as others). Tuition alone at many medical schools can be close to or more than $20,000 per year, which, while expensive, is still much cheaper than attending medical school outside Canada.

Once you're accepted to medical school (yay!), you will need to pay a deposit fee to hold your spot. This is not a huge amount relative to everything you have already paid and will pay, but it should still go on your budget list so you don't lose track of it. You may also be paying to update or fulfill first-aid and CPR credentials required by your medical school. In addition, you will need equipment to get you ready for the work you'll do as a medical student (check with your medical school: the list of equipment often includes a stethoscope, reflex hammer, tuning fork, and pen light, among other things). Of course, you'll need somewhere to live, and food to eat, and you will need to pay for books and tuition.

Three-year programs versus four-year programs

One way to potentially reduce your medical-school costs is to opt for a three-year program (very few schools offer these). A three-year program may save you nearly a year of tuition, living expenses, and lost wages. Students in three-year programs do not have summer breaks after their first and second year. Instead, they have a short couple of weeks before they start their next year. Currently, three-year programs are available at McMaster University and the University of Calgary.

Working versus not working during summers

Medical students do not get long summer breaks. The breaks are typically two months, and many students use their breaks for research,

---

EXERCISE: BUDGETING FOR MEDICAL-SCHOOL COSTS

Build a budget chart for medical-school costs. This helps you plan, and it's part of becoming an informed candidate that stands out.

In a column, make a list of the following items:

Deposit to hold acceptance spot

First-aid and CPR training or updating

Equipment (stethoscope, etc.: check the requirements of your medical school)

Books

Tuition fees (itemize each year)

Summer costs

Observerships (travel, accommodation, etc.)

Other (e.g., wedding, parental leave, sick leave)

After each item, describe its potential cost, your budget for it, and the date when you need to pay for it.

observerships (where you shadow physicians), travel, or medical volunteering. Unless your program doesn't allow it, you could theoretically get paid work during these breaks to offset the cost of your studies. If you have the option, you might consider the career value of this work opportunity and aim for something that not only lets you earn money, but also helps you with your next application process— applying for residency.

Scholarships and subsidies

Once you're accepted to medical school, you may qualify for financial help. For example, many medical schools have supportive alumni who have established funds to help students defray the high cost of medical-school tuition. I have heard that at one school a third of students receive full tuition assistance, a third receive partial tuition assistance, and only a third pay full tuition.

The Ontario Medical Student Bursary Fund is another avenue to pursue. This fund offers general assistance (given to students in greatest financial need at each Ontario medical school), named bursaries (check this list to see if you qualify because of your home location, intended practice location, and more) and elective bursaries (to help mitigate the costs of doing clinical electives during medical school). Other provinces may have similar assistance for medical students, so check in your jurisdiction.

Check with local community organizations such as Rotary International and with large corporations: these sometimes offer funding for specific employee groups or career goals.

Once you graduate, you may want to explore programs that help recruit and retain physicians to underserved areas of Canada. These come with financial incentives, and many provinces have them. (For more information, search *physician retention programs* with the name of a province or territory.)

PART II

APPLICATION ELEMENTS
AND HOW TO SHINE

*Read this section if you are preparing to
apply in the next couple of years.*

6

Application elements in context

When and where to apply

Some of the most common questions students ask include, Where should I apply? When should I apply? (And, when is the best time for me to apply?)

The answer to these questions depends on several factors, some of which are fixed, and others of which are in your control.

First, let's quickly review how the application process works in Canada.

The application process in Canada

ONTARIO: A CENTRALIZED PROCESS

Ontario has the largest number of medical schools (six) of any province in Canada, and applicants do not have to be Ontario residents to apply. Ontario medical schools mostly offer English-only programs: the University of Ottawa is the exception. Each school assesses you in the language of the program to which you apply. You might consider applying to:

- McMaster University (Hamilton): English program
- Northern Ontario School of Medicine (Sudbury): English program
- Queen's University (Kingston): QuARMS or regular programs in English

- University of Ottawa (Ottawa): French or English programs
- University of Toronto (Toronto): English program
- Western University (London): English program

You should visit each school's website for information about their program and application process, but, when you apply, the process is centralized through the Ontario Medical School Application Service (OMSAS), which is part of the Ontario Universities' Application Centre (OUAC) website. Even before you apply to medical school, you can find a lot of information on this site. I encourage you to read through it for a sense of what you'll need, when and if you decide to apply to any Ontario schools.

Some medical schools in Ontario have more than one campus, which is something else to consider when you apply (e.g., McMaster University has medical-school campuses in Hamilton, Niagara, and Waterloo).

OTHER PROVINCES: AN INDIVIDUAL PROCESS

Most medical schools outside Ontario reserve the majority of their spots for residents of their province. If you are applying to schools outside your home province (other than Ontario), check each year for the number of spots open to nonresidents. This will factor into your decision to apply. Most medical schools are unilingual (English or French), but some allow you to study in either official language. Again, each school assesses you in the language of the program to which you apply. You might consider applying to:

- Dalhousie University (Halifax, Nova Scotia): English program
- McGill University (Montreal, Quebec): English or French programs
- Memorial University (St. John's, Newfoundland): English program
- Université Laval (Quebec City, Quebec): French program
- Université de Montréal (Montreal, Quebec): French program
- Université de Sherbrooke (Sherbrooke, Quebec): French program
- University of Alberta (Edmonton, Alberta): English program
- University of British Columbia (Vancouver, British Columbia): English program
- University of Calgary (Calgary, Alberta): English program

- University of Manitoba (Winnipeg, Manitoba):
  English program
- University of Saskatchewan (Regina, Saskatchewan):
  English program

Despite the "odds" favouring home-province applicants to these schools, don't dismiss applying just because you're a nonresident. I worked with an Ontario student who applied to the University of British Columbia in a year when it had single-digit spots available to out-of-province applicants. I asked whether she really wanted to spend the money and effort to apply there, with so little chance of success. But, she was extremely enthusiastic about their program, and, in the end, she was one of the few students from her province accepted that year.

I encourage you to be realistic about the schools you apply to: make sure you meet the application requirements After that though, maybe you should close your ears to any naysayers, and apply where you want to attend and live.

Because medical-school applications are so competitive, many students apply everywhere and anywhere they can, simply to get in. While it's important to be realistic and apply broadly enough to give yourself the best chance, low-quality or inappropriate applications won't help you. In fact, they are a waste of money and effort.

When thinking about where to apply, consider:

- where you qualify as a resident
- at which schools you meet or exceed the requirements
- in which language or languages you are able to study
- how much time you can invest in each application
- what you can afford to pay in application fees
- where you want to live for the next three or four years (note that some medical schools have more than one campus—e.g., the University of British Columbia has academic campuses in Kelowna, Prince George, Vancouver, and Victoria)

Admission dates and strategies

The basics of when to apply vary by school. To my knowledge, medical schools in Canada all have September admission and start dates (unlike many schools in the Caribbean, for example, which have three admissions per year). You will likely apply in the year preceding the year you wish to be admitted, on the assumption that you will have completed any requirements for admission before dates determined by the program.

In Ontario, the OMSAS admission date for the past number of years has been October 1. You need to have created an account in the OMSAS system by mid-September to be able to apply. Always check to ensure that this is still the case.

Outside Ontario, deadlines are generally also during the autumn of the year preceding the year you wish to attend medical school.

As you are planning when to apply, be sure to also check MCAT release dates (i.e., the last date you can write the MCAT and still have it included in that year's application).

WHEN SHOULD *YOU* APPLY?

Once you have the general timelines in hand, the next question is, When is the best time for **you** to apply? As part of your decision-making process, you may want to ask yourself:

Do I meet or exceed the minimum criteria for each school to which I will apply?

Will I have an (excellent) MCAT score I can use by the time I apply?

Do my extracurricular and other activities clearly demonstrate the qualities medical schools want?

Do I have the time and money to submit high-quality applications now? How many do I have the time and money for?

Do I feel like I'm ready?

You may also need to consider or seek advice about:

- completing more courses before applying, to mitigate any blips in your GPA
- repeating the MCAT to try to better your score
- bolstering your autobiographical sketch, CV, or résumé—in general or in specific areas
- choosing more undergraduate work versus choosing graduate school as a next possible step
- improving your knowledge about what physicians do, so you are certain *you* want to do it and can communicate an informed choice

YEAR-BY-YEAR STRATEGIES

DURING HIGH SCHOOL

Keep in mind prerequisite courses required by many medical schools.

Talk to a guidance counsellor about your goals for medicine.

Become involved, or stay involved, in your school and larger community.

Save names and contact information for people who can verify your activities.

Investigate all kinds of career options, within medicine and outside it.

Keep an activities portfolio (it will help you with your auto-biographical sketch, CV, or résumé later).

Test out whether other careers, besides physician, might fit your goals. **Why *this* job?**

DURING FIRST-YEAR UNIVERSITY

Choose courses that interest you (you'll tend to do better).

Keep in mind prerequisite courses required by many medical schools.

Talk to an academic advisor in your faculty to find out how best to integrate prerequisites for medical school into your degree program.

Adapt to university while trying to stay involved in your community.

Keep your marks as high as you can, but realize it's only one year.

Balance work and school.

Investigate all kinds of career options, within medicine and outside it.

Keep an activities portfolio (it will help you with your auto-biographical sketch, CV, or résumé later).

Test out: **Why this job?**

DURING SECOND-YEAR UNIVERSITY

Research medical schools, including their admission require-ments and histories.

Check dates for writing the MCAT (consider writing it during or after your second year).

Decide on your MCAT study strategy: Will self-study or a course work best for you?

Start to gather references (e.g., get to know one or more of your professors, if you are in large classes).

Assess where you're at with prerequisites.

Start to get more specific about backup plans.

Organize job shadowing and information interviews.

Go to medical school websites and review detailed application information.

Develop an application budget.

Investigate application financial assistance.

Balance school and other parts of your life, and contribute to the broader community.

Assess your activities: Where do you want to focus or add variety? What about pursuing a leadership role in one activity?

Narrow down your answer: **Why this job?**

DURING THIRD- OR FOURTH-YEAR UNIVERSITY (OR FINAL YEAR)

Budget time, effort, money, and stress for the application process.

Write the MCAT during or after your third year (choose from test dates).

Approach your references: help them to help you.

Develop your application strategy (where to apply, how many applications in total).

Assess your candidacy and write applications.

Assess whether you fit any of the special categories for admission.

Complete your autobiographical sketch, CV, or résumé, and track down verifiers.

Organize transcripts.

Research areas of interest within the role of physician (i.e., specialties that interest you).

Have other people review your application.

Give yourself a break every once in a while—you deserve it!

Develop a travel budget for interviews and investigate financial assistance.

Revisit: **Why this job?** Show informed choice and a backup plan.

IF YOU'RE A GRADUATE STUDENT OR GRADUATING STUDENT

Check prerequisites to ensure you meet the most-current criteria.

Confirm possible additional required application documentation.

Confirm your MCAT scores are still valid, or rewrite the MCAT.

Meet, and keep in touch with, referees and verifiers.

Review your activities and reflect on patterns, strengths, and weaknesses.

Make decisions about whether and how to build on your activities while waiting to apply: if you're not working or studying, keep building experience.

Continue to be involved in your community (consider aiming for diversity or a leadership element).

Know that your undergraduate marks are still a major factor.

Follow final-year prep guidelines plus supplementary application information for graduate students.

STRATEGY EXAMPLES

I have worked with a lot of students applying to medical school. Each student is different, with decisions to make that are uniquely their own. Many students, however, face similar scenarios in deciding when to apply for medical school. Here are three common scenarios.

STUDENT 1

This student is currently in September of the third year of her undergraduate program. Her grades are strong, and she wrote the MCAT last summer and has her (strong) score. She wants to apply now so she can start medical school in what would have been her fourth year of undergrad.

Considerations

- Applying during the third year of her program means she will only be able to apply to medical schools that accept students without a four-year degree. However, this cuts down on the number of applications she can make, and so the expense and work of doing applications and interviews.
- Applying during third year means she has completed only two years and a bit of university work. Is she sure she meets the minimum credit requirement for each place she plans to apply? Also, her GPA will include only those two years. Many students have grades, especially from first-year university, that might bring down their GPA. Will her GPA be competitive, with fewer later grades to mitigate these blips?
- She will be younger than many in the applicant pool, so she will need to scrutinize her autobiographical sketch, CV, or résumé to ensure she has evidence that demonstrates the qualities sought by medical schools.
- If accepted, she will start medical school on the early side, getting to her dream career that much sooner, if all goes well.

STUDENT 2

This student is in his fourth year of an undergraduate degree. He has three grades in the low seventies from his early university years. His MCAT score is pretty strong. He has been very involved with student government and charitable organizations throughout high school and university, and feels that his extracurricular activities are impressive. He wants to apply to medical school during his fourth year, so he won't have a gap between the time he finishes his degree and the time he starts medical school.

Considerations

- Applying during fourth year means he should be able to apply to all medical schools, based on that element of their criteria.
- Because he is applying in his fourth year, his application will include grades from only his first three years of university. This means his lowest grades (from his first year) will likely have a bigger impact on his GPA than if he waited and applied after completing his fourth year (it is common for your grades to improve consistently after your first year in university).

Applying with grades that drag down his overall GPA might mean he will have difficulty being competitive at some medical schools, depending on the applicant pool that year.

- Will his strong extracurricular activities mitigate his lower GPA? He needs to read medical-school websites thoroughly to get a sense of this. He should consider contacting medical schools directly, to clarify whether they review extracurricular activities at the same time they review GPA and MCAT scores—or whether he must get through those gauntlets first, before they will see this other information.

- He should seek out schools that make allowances for lower grades (e.g., in the past, the University of Toronto has allowed applicants to leave their lowest three grades out of their cumulative GPA; Queen's University has calculated GPA from the last two years of an undergraduate degree if candidates didn't meet the minimum on their full degree). If he meets their criteria, perhaps he should apply there.

- If accepted, he can start medical school the year after he graduates from his first degree.

STUDENT 3

This is the same student as in the second scenario, except now he is in the year past graduation (or possibly a graduate student). He did not get accepted to medical school last year, when he applied. He also didn't receive any interviews.

Considerations

- Does missing out on interviews point to any particular part of his application that needs improvement?

- He will now have all his undergraduate grades. Will this boost his cumulative GPA? Does this encourage him to reapply, if he feels his GPA was a possible area of weakness?

- If his cumulative GPA has improved, due to the extra grades he can submit, does this expand where he can apply?

- If his GPA or MCAT score still need improvement to be competitive, does he wish to take steps to add additional undergraduate courses to his transcript or retake the MCAT? If he's a graduate student, which schools (if any) offer graduate students a slight GPA boost (or other boost)?

- How many times will he reapply to medical school before giving up?
- If accepted, he can start medical school the following year.

ASK YOURSELF

When to apply is a very personal decision and only you can make the right decision for yourself. Whatever you choose, I encourage you to think about the questions below. My observation, from working with thousands of students over the years, is that students who have thought about these questions tend to be most satisfied with their outcomes.

What is the balance of quantity versus quality for me?

If I apply to many places, will I feel that I submitted high-quality, realistic applications?

If I apply to only a few places, will I feel that I missed opportunities?

What strategy will help me decide what to do next, if and when I am accepted or rejected?

If I apply to places that reject me, will it help me figure out what to do next or whether to reapply?

If I apply to a place I don't really want to live and that's the one place I am accepted, what will I do?

How medical schools evaluate you

I do not speak for medical schools, but I have worked with thousands of students, helping them strategize about the elements of their applications and interviews. Strategizing involves "thinking like a medical school": How does each element help a medical school assess you, the candidate? This can push you to ensure that you are providing medical schools with the information and insights that are most useful to your candidate profile and their decision-making process.

The elements of evaluation

I discuss each application element in detail in the next chapters.

GRADE POINT AVERAGE AND PREREQUISITE COURSES

Academic excellence is a cornerstone of graduate education, and medical school is no exception. Every graduate program and medical school uses indicators

---

ASK YOURSELF

What does my transcript or GPA indicate about me?

such as GPA and performance in prerequisite courses to assess whether you have the building blocks of knowledge, or the potential to learn, that will help you succeed in their program.

MEDICAL COLLEGE ADMISSIONS TEST

Standardized tests such as the MCAT are another way that programs can assess your knowledge and academic capabilities. Most medical schools,

> **ASK YOURSELF**
> What might the way a medical school uses the MCAT hint about the information they're seeking?

if they consider the MCAT, use the whole thing. Others review only particular section scores.

AUTOBIOGRAPHICAL SKETCH, CURRICULUM VITAE, OR RÉSUMÉ

Grades and test scores alone do not provide medical schools enough information about you. The role of the autobiographical sketch, CV, or résumé is

> **ASK YOURSELF**
> How will my documents give insights into skills, experience, and qualities that medical schools evaluate?

to give them a fuller picture. This fuller picture is part of how they reduce the volume of applicants to a manageable number.

VERIFIERS

You will need to list people who can be contacted to vouch for the extracurricular activities you list in your autobio-

> **ASK YOURSELF**
> Who is in the best position to confirm each of my activities?

graphical sketch, CV, or résumé. You could think of verifiers as fraud deterrents—a way to ensure applicants are truthful and accurate about the activities they list.

COMPUTER-BASED ASSESSMENT FOR SAMPLING PERSONAL CHARACTERISTICS

A few medical schools use CASPer. I think more may move to it. It is a reasonably efficient way to assess a large number of applicants for their

> **ASK YOURSELF**
> Can I work through online scenarios in video and written format, giving effective, written answers in the time provided?

suitability for medicine, and to eliminate applicants with the least-best fit.

REFERENCES

Medical schools use references to help confirm or support other elements of your application. References provide written comments on your

ASK YOURSELF
What do others say about me? Do they think I am of good character and suitable for this career?

suitability and aptitude for medicine. They might also score you on qualities that medical schools seek.

SPECIAL-CATEGORY DOCUMENTS

Medical schools identify special categories for admission that target underrepresented groups in medicine. To apply under a special category, medical schools require documents

ASK YOURSELF
Do any special categories for admission apply to me? Do I wish to be considered under a special category?

to confirm that you identify as a member of a special category. In some cases, these documents may help reviewers understand more about your background.

INTERVIEWS

Interviews are time-consuming and labour intensive for medical schools to orchestrate. Why do they pour so much money and energy into them? Perhaps it's because interviews offer a way to assess candidates in real time.

ASK YOURSELF
As a candidate, can I establish connection and competency with a variety of people and situations? Can I communicate logically and with compassion?

What programs and degrees do medical schools accept?

Medical schools in Canada currently do not define what degree or degrees you should do before entering medicine. The majority of candidates

INSIDER INSIGHT
You can major in any degree program and apply to medical school.

with a student in film studies who wanted to spend his undergraduate time learning in a creative environment, with film production and directing as career options, but always with a view to becoming a doctor.

come from undergraduate or graduate programs in the sciences or health sciences, probably because these academic areas overlap with aspects of medicine and attract people with similar interests. I have worked with lots of these people. I have also worked with lots of undergraduate and graduate students from many other disciplines: engineering, philosophy, geography, psychology, fine arts, and more.

Certainly, the focus of your undergraduate degree is something to ponder, if you are in high school and contemplating university programs. In early university, it is still something to ponder: many students change their major a few times before settling on what works best for them.

There are lots of myths and rumours floating around about what I call "the hierarchy of degrees." Students sometimes get worked up about which degrees are viewed by medical schools as "best," as "harder," as "more elite."

In my view, your major is not that important. Medical schools accept students from any degree program. When I screened applicants for medical-school admissions, I often had no idea what degree program a candidate was doing—even at the interview stage. I interpret this as another sign (along with special-category admissions) that medical schools really are serious about wanting a diversity of backgrounds.

Do you love science? Do you love medieval history? Choose the program that you wish to pursue and that you feel will help best prepare you for a possible application to medical school (and other options). Which programs allow you to gather prerequisites for medicine that you might need?

Where do your academic skills lie? As much as the career practitioner in me wants to encourage students to "try things" and "expand your horizons" in university, if you are thinking about medical school, you need to make choices that

> **INSIDER INSIGHT**
> Given the heavy emphasis on cumulative, undergraduate grades for medical-school applications, you might want to choose a program strategically, to maximize your best academic performance.

maintain your grades. Even the odd elective course with an outlier grade can sometimes negatively affect your cumulative GPA.

What else might you want to do besides medicine? Consider programs that help leave doors open to other possible careers. I worked

When you transition to medical school, what programs do you think will prepare you best? Many arts and engineering students enter medical school and thrive in the program. Is it easier for students with an extensive background in science? This is a question for you to seek opinions about—but remember they are opinions only. Read what the medical schools say about preparation for their programs and weigh all this information against what you know about yourself.

There are also many applicants (and medical students) who have graduate or professional degrees such as master's degrees in pathology, epidemiology, or journalism, or doctorates in chemistry, pharmacy, optometry, or nursing—and many, many more. Medical schools heavily emphasize undergraduate grades, but they still accept students who pursue graduate school in related and non-related fields.

Considering all of the above, choose the program that best suits you.

How do medical schools view the university you are coming from?

As with degree programs, myths and rumours circulate about what I call "the hierarchy of schools," and students sometimes get worked up about which universities are viewed by medical schools as "best," as "harder," as "more elite."

In Canada, accredited universities don't suffer the reputational peaks and valleys that tend to rank universities in the United States. I believe every medical school in Canada has students from a cross-section of universities. Of course, students at particular universities and in particular programs may be more inclined to apply to medical school—which may have an impact on the number of students from that university at a given school. Students may also apply to medical schools that are geographically close to them and for which they meet the geographical residency criteria, and this may affect the number of students from particular universities at particular medical schools.

ONE SCHOOL'S STATISTICS

For the last couple of years, Dr. Anthony Sanfilippo, associate dean of Undergraduate Medical Education at Queen's University, has posted a blog revealing the composition of the incoming medical-school class. He has commented on how qualified and how academically diverse the classes are. (Search *Queen's undergraduate school of medicine blog* to see Dr. Sanfilippo's posts.)

INSIDER INSIGHT
Dr. Sanfilippo's 2017 blog post about the incoming class of 2021 reveals the wide variety of degree programs and universities from which the class hails.

If you look up this post or other lists of successful medical-school applicants, remember that these lists show students who happened to apply and get accepted in a particular year. Your university or program may not appear on the list, but that doesn't mean you are in the wrong university or degree.

What else do medical schools evaluate?

NONACADEMIC QUALITIES

Here is a list of qualities that medical schools tend to look for in their applicants. I compiled this list from medical-school statements about admission criteria. It may not fit perfectly with the particular criteria of the schools you apply to, which vary from year to year in any case. So check: do your own research. This list aims to give you an idea of skills, experience, and characteristics you may need to demonstrate.

Commitment and achievement

Problem-solving

Critical thinking

Informed choice

Self-directed learning

Scientific reasoning

Ability to function as a team player

Sensitivity to the needs of others

Adaptability, and ability to cope with stress

Interest in living and working with underserved populations

Interest in cross-cultural experiences

Involvement in volunteer work and extracurricular activities

EXERCISE: CHART YOUR FIT

You could use the list I compiled as a starting point for building, or adding to, your autobiographic sketch, CV, or résumé. Make a chart, with each item on the list in a column. Next to each item, describe evidence from your life that demonstrates the skill, experience, or quality.

Refine this list based on particular criteria of the schools to which you apply, in the year you apply.

INSIDER INSIGHT

You also might want to research the CanMeds framework from the Royal College of Physicians and Surgeons of Canada. (Use *CanMeds framework* as the search term in your browser.)

While I am not aware of any official evaluation of medical-school applicants based on this framework, I believe it offers another useful way to think about your own qualities and candidacy.

CLUSTERS AND ACTIVITY TYPES

Some medical schools ask you to comment on, or refine, your list of activities against specific criteria. This requires you to reflect on your activities and make decisions. Here are some examples of criteria:

- The University of Toronto in 2018 grouped and assessed candidates' activities in four "clusters": a professional cluster; a cluster covering communication, collaboration, and leadership; an advocate cluster; and a scholar cluster.
- The University of British Columbia in 2018 asked applicants to choose from among their activities those experiences that fit specific "activity types," including leadership, service ethic, capacity to work with others, diversity of experience, and high performance in an area of human endeavour.

As you engage in and track your activities, I encourage you not simply to "collect" them. Take time to reflect on them, including your accomplishments, your learning and growth, and your challenges. If you plan to apply to specific medical schools, you might want to make a chart that helps you allocate activities according to their criteria (e.g., the clusters of the University of Toronto or the activity types of the University of British Columbia). This can help you assess where you might need to undertake a new activity, before you apply.

ASSESSING THE COMPETITIVENESS OF YOUR NONACADEMIC QUALITIES

Medical schools are usually quite clear about the non-academic qualities they are seeking in their candidates. Be sure to consult their websites and any application guides they offer.

In addition, reflect on your extracurricular activities as you consider what to join, stop, and start. Think about the patterns they form, and what these patterns might tell someone about your suitability for medicine, and your ability not only to get into medical school, but graduate from it.

ASK YOURSELF

Do I stop and start things?

Do I spread myself too thin?

Can I manage several things at the same time?

Do I attend school and do little or nothing else?

Have I seen a problem and contributed to bettering it?

Have I been exposed to a variety of people and situations?

7

Grade point average

Medical schools receive thousands of applications every year for a relatively small number of total spots. They have the luxury, in a way, of starting with the strongest academic candidates. We can debate how fair that is, but medical schools are unlikely to change this strategy. Why would they? The strongest academic candidates generally succeed at medical school, and GPA is a way to assess a huge number of applicants in a straightforward and efficient manner.

For example, say a medical school receives 12,000 applications, from which it might choose 500 applicants to interview for the 100 spots it has available. Instead of having to read and possibly interview 12,000 people, it can simply identify the top 500 GPAs (possibly in tandem with MCAT scores) and then, boom, interview those 500 people.

This does not mean that medical schools ignore the parts of your application that describe your extracurricular activities, or that they place no value on interviews. It does mean that medical schools have such a high volume of candidates that they may not look at "the rest of you" until you've first made it through the GPA (and, possibly, MCAT score) gauntlet.

Medical schools usually state only a minimum GPA requirement in their instructions for application (e.g., 3.0 on a 4-point scale). However, this minimum does not usually reflect the current applicant pool (e.g., the average GPA of the top 500). The average GPA of the applicant pool varies from year to year, but the average is often high (e.g., 3.96+ out of 4.0). A few medical schools post the average GPA of their incoming class. Remember, this is an average and does not necessarily reflect the uniqueness of each applicant. It is perhaps for this reason that many medical schools do **not** post this statistic—they want to encourage a broad candidacy, because there are exceptions to every rule.

An extremely high GPA across a large number and variety of undergraduate courses demonstrates your academic abilities, and also your ability to manage a lot of course work (many medical schools have a minimum course load requirement in your undergraduate degree) with other priorities such as working, volunteering, participating in sports, and contributing to your community.

The emphasis on GPA for medical-school admission might have another driver, too—the idea that knowledge helps keep patients safe. Medical schools could argue that they need to recruit candidates with high motivation for academic excellence because the grading system in medical school may be only pass/fail. Nobody wants a mediocre surgeon or family doctor, do they?

I have spoken with many students who are discouraged by the high GPA and seemingly blemish-free academic record they believe medical schools require. They argue that they are young. They are figuring out university still. They are going through all kinds of life transitions—moving away from home, new mental illness, roommates, figuring out university learning styles, and buying their own toilet paper. Isn't it natural that some academic issues would happen?

I completely agree. However, I can also understand how logistics, for now, continue to make GPA a key piece of information for medical schools.

Variations on calculating grade point average

Most medical schools in Canada require you to submit your cumulative GPA. Medical schools have instructions about how to calculate what that figure is. The instructions differ from place to place and possibly even from year to year, so be sure to check the most current instructions.

Ontario

We'll start with Ontario, because all spots in Ontario medical schools are open to all applicants in Canada. In other provinces, medical schools reserve most of their spots for residents of those provinces.

In Ontario, medical-school applications are centralized, and so is the process of calculating your GPA. Each course on your transcript is weighted with several credits (usually 1 for a half-year course, 2 for a full-year course). This means that a full-year course in which you did particularly well will—sort of—get counted twice. Unfortunately, it also means that a full-year course in which you did particularly poorly will also get counted twice.

OMSAS (the Ontario Medical School Application Service) has a table to help you calculate your cumulative GPA, according to the system your university uses for grading (e.g., a university may issue letter grades, or it may issue grades in percentages). The table is available online (use the search term *OMSAS GPA conversion*).

Two things to note about this table:

- Its order is **not** based on how "good" your undergraduate school is. Many students incorrectly assume that their school's row in the table somehow indicates the perceived reputation or quality of the university they attend. Rather, the position of your university in the table reflects the grading system at your university: the table groups like grading systems together. For example, if your university grades on a 4-point scale, it will appear in the same part of the table as other universities that grade this way.

- The table is somewhat imprecise, in my experience. Students report to me that the table doesn't deliver an exact cumulative GPA, which they find frustrating. They want an exact number to figure out if they are competitive. Given the large number of grading systems the table incorporates, it makes sense that the table can only get to a certain level of precision. If you have questions about what to do in your situation, check with OMSAS or your target medical schools to see what they recommend.

Outside Ontario

In other provinces, each school has a method for submitting or converting your cumulative GPA. This is also true for medical schools outside of Canada. You need to consult each medical school to find out about their process for submitting or converting your GPA.

Pay careful attention in these situations, so you don't waste opportunities by accidentally submitting to schools where your cumulative GPA misses the minimum requirement.

Some schools have a "forgiveness" element to their calculations. For example, University of Toronto has, in the past, allowed students to exclude the lowest three grades from their transcript, when submitting their cumulative GPA. Other schools only require you to submit the last fifteen courses you took. If you feel your GPA is "on the cusp," you might want to pay particular attention to these exceptions when you're considering where to apply.

INSIDER INSIGHT
Even if a medical school appears to use the same grading system as your university or as another medical school, it may use a different conversion process for your GPA. Always ask for the specific conversion process.

Strategies for converted grades

If you are applying in Ontario, or to a medical school that requires you to convert your university grades to a 4-point scale, minor variances in your grades can sometimes have a bigger impact on your cumulative GPA than you expected.

The closer your grades are to each other, the less variation you will tend to see when you convert them to a 4-point cumulative GPA.

For example, a grade of 68%, even when balanced with a grade of 98%, might cause a bigger drop in cumulative GPA than grades of 85% and 82%.

To help mitigate the odd lower grade, you can increase the total number of undergraduate courses you take. I discuss strategies to overcome a GPA that is holding you back in chapter 16.

TIPS FOR HIGH SCHOOL OR EARLY UNIVERSITY
If you are in high school and about to enter university, or if you are early in your first degree, aim to get grades that are high and "cluster" together.

The emphasis on undergraduate grades

The current climate at medical schools is that undergraduate grades are of primary and ongoing importance. Even if medical schools assess your application separate from the general applicant pool (e.g., if you are a graduate student), your undergraduate GPA still stands as a key element of the academic part of your application.

A small number of schools may afford you a very slight (emphasis on *very*) GPA boost if you are a graduate student, but in my experience it usually hasn't been enough to positively impact those students who need it. But, if you are already in graduate school, be sure to check, in case it does help you.

What do your grades say about you?

Ideally, long before you apply to medical school, you will start looking at your grades to assess where they might need improvement. Many students I have worked with do this during the final year of their undergraduate degree, which is not ideal. We can come up with some strategies at that point, but it is easier to alter your course earlier in your university education. The earlier you start this process, the better.

EXERCISE: CHART YOUR GRADES

Try building a chart like the one that follows to help you track and assess your grades.

MEDICAL SCHOOL	PREREQUISITES: WHAT DO I NEED? WHEN WILL I FIT THEM IN?	GPA CALCULATION AT THIS SCHOOL	RED FLAGS IN MY TRANSCRIPT	NOTES

Atypical transcripts

I worked with a student who was diagnosed with leukemia during her second year of university. She left school for a period to get treatment and then tried to return in third year to get back on track with her studies. She suffered a relapse during third year and was unable to keep up with her studies. Her transcript was full of courses started and stopped, and in some cases not completed.

When she applied to medical school after she graduated from her undergraduate degree, she felt she was a strong candidate, in part because of her personal experience with illness and the health-care system. This experience was very well illustrated in the applications she prepared and, of course, she knew she could talk about it in interviews. However, there still remained the "problem" with her transcript. Would the longer-than-usual length of her undergraduate degree affect her transcript review? Would medical schools even see that detail, or would they simply see her cumulative GPA (which was in the lower ranges of excellent)?

She was applying in Ontario, so when filling out her autobiographical sketch, she included an entry in the "other" section that said something like, "Successfully treated for life-threatening disease during second- and third-year university." I believe she may have also consulted medical schools to ask whether she could or should include a letter, along with her transcript, outlining the reasons her transcript looked a bit different than the average candidate—with the emphasis placed on how she had successfully overcome these obstacles.

In any case, she was successful at getting interviews and is currently attending medical school.

Not making the cut on grades

GPA remains a key element in helping medical schools both assess candidacy and manage the large volume of applications they receive.

In my experience, students who don't meet the GPA cut are **not** mediocre or just "good" students: they are excellent students. If you don't get into medical school when you apply, try not to view it as an academic failure. You may need to apply more than once. You may need to assess whether there are things you can do to improve the GPA you submit. However, with the likely strong GPA you already possess, you have many other academic and nonacademic career options available to you—so consider these. And do your homework: as long as you meet a medical school's minimum criteria, you are eligible to apply. Decide when and if it makes sense for you to do so.

8

Medical College Admission Test

The MCAT helps medical schools assess whether you have the pre-requisite knowledge and aptitudes to succeed in medical school. In my view, it also allows medical schools to deal efficiently with a large volume of applications: assessing something quantitative, such as a grade or score, is more straightforward than assessing something qualitative, such as compassion or community mindedness.

The MCAT is a standardized test. This means it is "the same" for everyone, which makes an MCAT score easy to compare to other MCAT scores. This is different than a grade in Biology 30, for example: although many people take this "same" course, Biology 30 grades reflect a variety of provincial curricula, classrooms, schools, teachers, and grading schemes. In a standardized test, such as the MCAT, everyone engages the same content for the same purpose, and they are ostensibly graded in the same way.

If you have always lived in Canada or have only applied (or plan to apply) to Canadian programs, you may be less familiar with stan-dardized tests than other students. Unlike students who apply to university in the United States, for example—who write standard-ized admission tests (SATs)—most students in Canada have never been required to write a standardized test. A few graduate programs in Canada review this type of admissions criteria, and standard-ized tests are the norm for students applying to professional facul-ties such as law school (LSAT), clinical psychology or epidemiology

(GRE), pharmacy (PCAT), dentistry (DAT), optometry (OAT), and business administration (GMAT).

Most medical schools in Canada and the United States use part or all of the MCAT in their application criteria. The MCAT is a multiple-choice, timed exam designed to assess your skills in critical thinking and problem solving, and concepts in natural science, behavioural science, and social science. You can't write just one section of the MCAT, so even if a medical school reviews only one section as part of their process and you are applying only there, you still need to write the entire exam.

The MCAT is coordinated by the Association of American Medical Colleges (AAMC). You register for the MCAT with the AAMC, and the AAMC releases your score to the medical schools to which you apply. The AAMC has information on its website about taking the MCAT and provides useful orientation (use the search term *AAMC taking the MCAT*).

Since 2015, when the MCAT underwent a major overhaul, writing the test takes the best part of a day (instead of its former half day) and includes the following sections:

- Chemical and Physical Foundations of Biological Systems
- Critical Analysis and Reasoning Skills (CARS)
- Biological and Biochemical Foundations of Living Systems
- Psychological, Social, and Biological Foundations of Behaviour

Depending on your academic program, you might feel more or less comfortable, at first glance, with these topics. If you are considering a career in medicine and planning to write the MCAT—even if you are in high school or just starting in university—think about how you can best prepare yourself to succeed with the MCAT's topics and the MCAT's testing environment.

Preparing for the MCAT

High school and university courses that can help

I have heard MCAT course instructors comment that many of the science sections on the MCAT mostly engage high school material. If this is true, you may wish to take some courses related to MCAT topics in grade 11 or 12. In addition to helping you with the MCAT, these courses could be prerequisites for university science courses—which may also help you prepare for the MCAT.

An MCAT course instructor also told me that taking a first-year university psychology course could be good preparation for the section of the MCAT on psychological, social, and biological foundations of behaviour. I have also heard comments that university humanities and arts courses can help prepare for the CARS section of the test. Many students anecdotally comment that taking the MCAT shortly after they completed a university biochemistry course was a good strategy, because biochemistry was still fresh in their minds. Many science students comment that they are the most nervous about the CARS section and the section on foundations of behaviour—some students feel comfortable with the material they find in sample questions, but worry about the timing involved in the actual test.

Some students choose to include courses relevant to topics on the the MCAT (e.g., psychology, biology, physics) in their university work. They do this even if these courses are not part of their program, and even if the courses are not prerequisites for medical school. Other students can't fit in extra courses like this, or decide they prefer to prepare for some MCAT topics through self-study (e.g., books or courses). Whatever the rumours and advice, you need to work out the best plan for you, depending on how you learn, how independently you learn, and how much time and money you have for studying. There is no "best" way and students use a variety of strategies for success.

Prep courses versus books

Many organizations are lined up to help you prepare for the MCAT (and take your money.) I am not advocating that you use any of them. However, some students find some or all of the following useful in their preparations:

- taking courses during high school and university that cover MCAT topics
- self-study with MCAT books (buying or borrowing MCAT study books to prepare)
- courses (online or in-person courses that guide you through MCAT preparation with instructions, practice exams, and more)
- tutoring, offered privately or through a course, with a focus on particular MCAT topics (which might include topics you

anticipate having trouble with, or in which you have already received lower-than-optimal grades)

Think about the type of learner you are. Would a structured, guided approach with homework and practice exams be most effective for you? If yes, consider a course. Would working through structured materials and practice exams at your own pace work better? If yes, consider self-study with MCAT-specific materials. I also know students who have created their own course of study, using materials they sourced themselves, who have done well on the exam. So, self-structured self-study is also an option. (Students who choose this option often borrow MCAT-specific books for the practice exams they contain.)

All methods work effectively for students. What will work effectively for you?

EXERCISE: CHART YOUR MCAT PREPARATION

Build a chart, like the one that follows , to figure out your best route through preparing for the MCAT.

MCAT SECTIONS	WHAT PREREQUISITES MIGHT HELP ME?	WHAT OTHER RESOURCES MIGHT HELP ME (E.G., STUDY BOOKS, COURSES)?	PRACTICE EXAMS: WHEN WILL I WRITE THEM?	NOTES
Chemical and Physical Foundations of Biological Systems	In high school			
	In university			
Critical Analysis and Reasoning Skills (CARS)	In high school			
	In university			
Biological and Biochemical Foundations of Living Systems	In high school			
	In university			
Psychological, Social, and Biological Foundations of Behaviour	In high school			
	In university			

Factors, besides learning style, that may affect your decision include:

- the location and availability of materials and courses
- timing that works for you
- structure versus flexibility in schedule and approach
- cost (including costs from different MCAT-preparation companies)
- recommendations from other students

Cost

In 2018, the basic cost to write the MCAT was $315 USD. You incur additional costs if you register late, change your registration, or require testing at an international test site (Canada is not considered international).

When to write

The MCAT had thirty test dates available in Canada in 2018—and a similar number in past years—so, choose the timing that works best for you. Keep in mind that most students prefer to write during the summer months, so summer test dates book very quickly. (The MCAT posts more test dates for the summer to help compensate for this.)

I have heard students mention that taking the MCAT during the academic year helped them approach their preparation for it as simply another course. Still others prefer to focus on it during the summer and then write it before going back to school in the fall. Some students take it after second year or close to finishing a particularly relevant course (e.g., biochemistry). As long as your MCAT score will still be valid by the time you apply to medical school, when you take it is up to you.

MCAT score validity

Many medical schools will not accept an MCAT score that is more than three years old, so factor this into your planning.

If you are not writing the MCAT and applying to medical school in quick succession, remember to review carefully the last test date you can write to ensure your MCAT score is valid for the application deadlines you need to meet.

Medical schools usually allow you to release your score to them, once you receive it, if you are writing the MCAT close to their submission dates. However, if you are in this situation, you won't know whether your MCAT score meets their minimum criteria, or how competitive it is, before you pay to apply to medical schools.

> **INSIDER INSIGHT**
> Some students write the MCAT in September. This means that— at least for medical schools in Ontario, where the application deadline is October 1—they will be submitting applications without knowing their MCAT scores, because MCAT scores normally take one month to be processed.

How many times you can write (really)

Currently, the AAMC allows students to write the MCAT a maximum of three times per year.

As an advisor, I suggest considering that option carefully. Many, many students write the MCAT twice (whether or

> **INSIDER INSIGHT**
> Be intentional and strategic about writing the MCAT.

not in the same year), and, at least in my experience, twice doesn't appear to disadvantage them in their application process.

I never suggest that a student "throw away" an MCAT opportunity (e.g., "I think I'll try the MCAT next week and see how it goes, because I can always rewrite it"). Every MCAT score might become part of your application record.

If you are writing the MCAT more than once, be prepared to defend your decision. Wanting to improve your initial score— whether to meet minimum criteria or to increase your chances of success—can be a valid defence. Still, think about how you would defend subsequent attempts, and how much more challenging that defence might become with successive attempts (three, four, five).

Medical schools vary in how they ask you to report repeated MCAT scores. Some want only the latest score (this can be disappointing, if you don't do as well on a subsequent writing), or the highest score, or a combination of scores. Be sure to consider these differences when deciding whether to rewrite.

ASK YOURSELF

The following questions help build a strategy around rewriting the MCAT.

Do I have enough time and capacity to prepare for a rewrite, so that I can post a better outcome?

Have I done research to assess the likelihood of posting a better outcome (i.e., has repeat testing worked for other students)?

Are there particular elements of the test that I can improve? For example: If running out of time was a factor on previous attempts, how can I practise timed writings before the next exam? If particular sections gave me trouble, how can I devote extra study time to those topics?

Is a better score required before I can realistically apply or have a competitive application? Could I apply with my current score and, in a sense, get my feedback from the medical schools' response?

Does the additional, potentially better score offset the number of times I've written the test? (Can I defend rewriting?)

Whether to write

Some students choose to apply to medical schools that do not require the MCAT. While this greatly limits where you can apply, it is still an option in Canada. Most candidates choose to write the MCAT so that they can maximize the scope of their applications. If you worry that your GPA is a bit iffy, the MCAT can provide an additional, quantitative way for you to demonstrate aptitudes desired by medical schools. Ideally, both your GPA and MCAT scores will be strong enough to allow you to apply to several medical schools, meeting or exceeding their basic criteria.

How your MCAT will be assessed

The process of reviewing your MCAT score (where required) varies by medical school. Medical schools outline what scores they require from applicants. Often, this includes a minimum total score as well as minimum section scores. If your total score is great, but one of your section scores doesn't meet the minimum, your MCAT score might not meet the minimum criteria. A couple of schools review only one section of the MCAT—in these cases, your total score isn't a factor at all.

As with GPA, schools may state a minimum required MCAT score, which may or may not reflect the realities of the current applicant pool (i.e., the minimum score they state may be much lower than the scores of most applicants). However, if you meet the minimum, you are eligible to apply. Having said that, strive for your highest score possible to solidify that part of your application.

Accommodations

As with many other types of exams, and other parts of medical-school admissions, you may require accommodations for a disability to complete the MCAT. Since the test is American, this may be governed by the Americans with Disabilities Act, which may, in some cases, differ from policies you have experienced in Canada. There is detailed information on the MCAT website about how to request accommodations for the exam (search with the term *AAMC MCAT exam with accommodations*).

## 9

Autobiographical sketch, curriculum vitae, or résumé

What this application element is for and what to include

Even though academic abilities are a key part of the basic criteria for assessing medical students, they are not the only qualities that help to predict a good medical student, resident, or physician. So, medical schools evaluate candidates' nonacademic qualities for that reason. In addition, this assessment helps pare down the number of qualified applicants: even after the GPA and MCAT review stage, this number generally still far exceeds the spots available at any particular medical school.

To evaluate nonacademic qualities, medical schools ask for supplemental materials in the form of an autobiographical sketch, CV, or résumé. The focus of this application element varies by medical school and it is continually evolving. In my view, it evolves because medical schools scrutinize the benefits they get from the immense time involved in assessing these supplemental materials—which requires individual, qualitative candidate review—and they make adjustments to close loopholes and refine processes that seem to yield the most suitable candidates.

Often, more than one person will be reviewing any supplemental materials you are asked to submit. As a medical-school admissions volunteer, I often screened the supplemental materials of twenty-five to thirty applicants, which was, of course, not nearly the total number of applicants that the medical school reviewed. You can imagine the workforce required to assess hundreds—potentially thousands—of candidates at this level. I have noticed that, in recent years, schools have considerably reduced the supplemental materials they require.

For example, each and every medical school used to ask for essays and responses to short-answer questions, in addition to an autobiographical sketch, CV, or résumé. Although a few schools still include these as part of their application process, most now request *only* an autobiographical sketch, CV, or résumé.

This, of course, delivers both good news and bad news. If you are a candidate who easily meets the quantitative part of applications with your GPA and MCAT score, then you might rejoice that very few applications require additional writing. If you are someone who is less sure about those quantitative elements, you might mourn the loss of more opportunities to demonstrate your other qualities.

Medical schools that have reduced the supplemental materials they require clearly have their reasons: maybe they have other ways to assess the nonacademic qualities of applicants, or they have found essays and short-answer questions less than insightful in the past, or they have decided to recruit fewer volunteers and staff for their applicant reviews. I suspect it is a combination of these and other reasons.

Some medical schools give feedback to applicants who are not invited to interviews: often the feedback says their supplemental materials were not competitive for the applicant pool. The strategies in this chapter aim to explain what medical schools assess through supplemental materials, and give you ideas for building and describing activities that will be helpful to your application and those who read your application.

Ontario

Ontario applications to medical school are centralized through OMSAS. You create and submit online a single autobiographical sketch: *all* the schools in Ontario to which you are applying receive this autobiographical sketch. This greatly maximizes efficiency for you as an applicant, but you also need to consider the focus of each school regarding this sketch when you are crafting this one document. (Check the requirements of each medical school to determine its focus.)

Graduate students applying in Ontario may be required to submit a CV, in addition to the autobiographical sketch.

The instructions for the autobiographical sketch require you to submit activities from age sixteen onwards. Currently, you have up to thirty-two "entries" in the sketch to write about your activities, each with a word limit. You do **not** need to fill all thirty-two entries (nor should you, necessarily). Naturally, the older you are when you apply to medical school, the more entries you may have and vice versa for younger applicants. Still, every applicant should think strategically about which activities to include. Review carefully what each school evaluates as you make decisions about what to keep and what to leave out.

The sketch comprises sections similar to a CV or résumé. However, it allows only the following, specific sections:[1]

(F) Formal Education

(E) Employment

(V) Volunteer Activities

(X) Extracurricular Activities

(A) Awards and Accomplishments

(R) Research

(O) Other

The instructions for the sketch advise you to include both structured and nonstructured experiences. For example, you may work with a local youth group once per week (structured) and you may help your grandma out after school (nonstructured). Both could be considered for inclusion on your document.

Here's an example of how a sketch might look:

#	CAT	DATE RANGE	DESCRIPTION	GEOGRAPHIC LOCATION
1	F	2014/09–2016/06	O.S.S.D., Nippissing Secondary School	North Bay, ON
2	F	2016/09–ongoing	BSc, Chemistry, Trent University	Peterborough, ON
3	F	2016/09–ongoing	BEd (concurrent), Queen's University	Kingston, ON
4	E	2017/05–2017/08	Oncology Research Asst, Toronto General Hospital	Toronto, ON

#	CAT	DATE RANGE	DESCRIPTION	GEOGRAPHIC LOCATION
5	V	2017/01– ongoing	Recreation Asst 3hrs/wk, Boys and Girls Club	Peterborough, ON
6	X	2016/09– ongoing	Varsity Rower @ 15–20 hrs/wk, Queen's University	Peterborough, ON
7	A	2013/04– 2013/07	3-mnth ed'l exchange (lived with host family)	Lyons, France
8	A	2016/09– 2017/06	Govnr General Award for Highest Average	North Bay, ON
9	R	2019/09– ongoing	4th yr thesis prjct: Effect of M&Ms on mice	Peterborough, Ontario
10	O	2014/05– ongoing	Family travel to 14 countries	Europe, Asia

Outside Ontario

Applications to medical schools outside Ontario are individual to each school. For supplemental materials, you may be asked to submit a résumé or CV. Although these two documents are technically different, in the context of a medical-school application they mean basically the same thing.

A résumé is usually a document you would use to apply for work or volunteering. Just like when you're applying for work or volunteering, a résumé for a medical-school application needs to consider its audience: What categories and information would be most relevant to that audience? Review what each medical school has asked you to include in your résumé or CV. Some schools may ask you to include particular sections or clusters of experiences. If they give no instructions, plan to cover at least the following categories of information:

- education
- awards and accomplishments
- work experience
- volunteer experience
- research experience (if applicable)
- extracurricular activities

You might consider restructuring this traditional list of categories into more targeted categories, such as those that follow. These restructured categories could include experiences from a variety of areas of your life, not just paid work.

- health-related experience
- community service experience
- science and laboratory experience
- leadership experience
- social justice experience

These are just examples of categories you could use. You may have a completely different list, or a longer or shorter list.

If you are a graduate student, you may be submitting something that looks a bit more like a CV. In addition to, or instead of, typical résumé categories, it might include (if applicable) categories such as:

- publications
- research funding
- poster presentations
- abstracts
- teaching experience
- other categories related to your scholarly experience (if applicable)

Building activities to include in this application element

Among the many nonacademic qualities medical schools seek in their applicants, I found the following from a recent look at medical-school admissions criteria:

Commitment and achievement

Problem-solving

Critical thinking

Informed choice

Self-directed learning

Scientific reasoning

Ability to function as a team player

Sensitivity to the needs of others

Adaptability, and ability to cope with stress

Interest in living and working with underserved populations

Interest in cross-cultural experiences

Involvement in volunteer work and extracurricular activities

INSIDER INSIGHT

As you live your life, and choose courses, programs, and schools, get involved and contribute to the community around you. Think about how what you are doing (and how you're doing it) demonstrates and builds skills that medical schools desire.

You might want to make a chart with these and additional qualities, and fill it in with examples that show how you demonstrate them (I also recommended this step, with this list of qualities, in chapter 6.)

Strategic involvement

Many students are extremely involved in volunteer and extracurricular activities during high school, while others are less so.

Often, students' volunteer and extracurricular activities are not quite as extensive in university as they are in high school, due to the increased academic workload, but students still need to demonstrate involvement with activities outside the classroom. Bearing in mind what medical schools say they are looking for, there are really no "right" or "wrong" activities to engage with. Choose what makes sense for you, your location, interests, and abilities, and your schedule. Think about how your activities relate to your future medical-school application and career. Then, keep half an eye on the overall patterns and messages that these might convey to someone reading your medical-school application, in the (perhaps distant) future. For example, I often ask students to reflect on whether they feel their activities help them demonstrate that:

- They can achieve high grades academically while also balancing other priorities.
- They see problems and seek to contribute to their solution.

TIPS FOR HIGH SCHOOL AND EARLY UNIVERSITY

If you think you may apply to medical school, consider scrutinizing your out-of-classroom activities to see if you should add to them or edit them. Consider the same scrutiny of activities in university.

ASK YOURSELF

Are there populations, issues, or subjects that grab my interest and that I could contribute to in some way?

Am I aware of a problem, need, or issue in my school, local community, or region that I could start something to address (if nothing already exists)?

What are the attributes (if any) of this activity that might help me decide whether I want to be a physician?

What is a realistic number of activities for me to manage, so that my grades don't suffer?

- They are developing and learning about themselves in a well-rounded way.

When considering "strategic" volunteering, you may want to think about what your activities say about your interests, your engagement with your community, your exploration of medicine as a profession, and your ability to achieve balance in your life.

Research

If you are an undergraduate student, you will likely not have much (if anything) to include in a "research" section of your autobiographical sketch, CV, or résumé. This is not unusual, but consider pursuing research opportunities if they present themselves, because research is an aspect of medical school and residency.

TIPS FOR HIGH SCHOOL AND EARLY UNIVERSITY

If you are in high school or early university, you may wish to seek out opportunities to engage with research (as a volunteer, subject, thesis project, observership, summer job), both to find out what it's all about and to show that this type of scholarly learning is something you have tried.

Don't worry too much if the research opportunities you encounter are not especially related to your possible interest areas in medicine. Exposure to the doldrums, methodologies, excitement, and environments of research seems to be valuable.

Volunteering and extracurricular activities

Whether you're still in high school or are already in university or doing graduate work, you will need to continue to show your desire to get involved with other people and your ability to balance competing priorities. It is normal to see candidates with a few activities that span multiple years, perhaps to the point of taking on positions of leadership.

For example, membership in a student group in year one might lead to a committee position in that same group in year two and three, and possibly a role in the group executive in year four.

Not every activity you participate in needs to (or should) look like this, but it's perhaps useful to show that you have committed to some activities in a longer-term way, and have sought opportunities to contribute in a variety of roles.

There will also likely be activities that you tried once, or for a period (e.g., one year), and, for whatever reason, didn't continue. I believe that this is normal and likely "acceptable," as long as it doesn't seem to form a big pattern in your history.

Other

Have you also included relevant, nonstructured activities? If you are applying with the online autobiographical sketch, does your "other" section loom empty? If you are submitting a CV or résumé, do you go beyond the traditional work, volunteer, and extracurricular activities to include experiences that have shaped you, taken significant time, and been a big part of your life? Think about these and other types of activities that might apply to you, such as:

- running several times a week, by yourself
- training for an event (athletic, arts, science, other)
- playing violin every day
- driving a neighbour to get groceries regularly
- helping with the family farm or business
- travelling with family or others
- living with an ill or differently abled sibling or relative
- overcoming an illness or disease yourself (use caution here— this might work for you or against you, so it's good to seek advice about if and how to include and describe this)

I once worked with a student who mentioned that she was having trouble coming up with the money to apply to medical school, because she and her family lived below the poverty line. She had not thought of including this information in her autobiographical sketch. In fact, this information highlighted important qualities about her, and also helped explain why her work category was so full and other categories (volunteer activities, extracurricular activities) slightly less so, compared to other candidates. She decided to include information about her financial situation, and I gave her feedback as she drafted and redrafted the it, until she felt happy with it.

Verifiers

For some applications, you need to provide verifiers for some or all of your activities. A verifier is a person who can confirm, when contacted, that you participated in an activity you describe. Meeting this requirement can be stressful for applicants who are only learning about it in late university or during graduate work, because activities from high school or even early university may have taken place a long time ago.

TIPS FOR HIGH SCHOOL AND EARLY UNIVERSITY

If you are reading this in high school, try to stay in touch with teachers, coaches, leaders, and others after you graduate, so that you know how to find them and can ask them to be verifiers.

If you are already in university or doing graduate work, you may have to track down people you used to know to ask them to be verifiers. That is also very normal—it just means that the "verifier step" may take more time and feel more stressful. If you can't list a required verifier for an activity, you may have to leave that activity out of your autobiographical sketch, CV, or résumé.

Quality versus quantity

While quantity helps with this application element, it is also important to consider quality.

Sometimes, the decision to include an activity revolves around how long you were involved in it, because long-

ASK YOURSELF

Why am I including a particular activity (if it's not compulsory)? How would I defend its place in my autobiographical sketch, CV, or résumé?

term involvement leads to in-depth connection. However, two-hour opportunities can also be extremely meaningful. It varies with each student, and it's up to you to decide what your activities demonstrate about you, and which ones merit inclusion in medical-school applications.

Be cautious about including every single thing you have done. Can you describe all those activities really well, so that they earn their place in your autobiographical sketch, CV, or résumé? Can you defend why they are there, if asked? Quantity does not necessarily beat quality.

Strategies for this element in high school, university, and beyond

High school

High school is a wonderful time to start getting a sense of what you really love to do and what you're good at. Here are some strategies that will help you build an autobiographical sketch, CV, or résumé for medical school:

- Choose activities that let you try out interests and build new skills. Don't censor yourself too much—simply allow yourself to participate in opportunities that appeal to you. This is a great strategy for this time in your life.

- Start a résumé file, perhaps both electronic and paper. If it's paper, put certificates and awards, diplomas, and letters of reference in it. Use your electronic file to build a basic résumé, which you can use to apply for work and volunteering, but that will also serve as a skeleton for your submission to medical school. A résumé file will help you keep track of dates and details associated with activities that, by the time you apply, may be some time ago.

- Consider taking on leadership roles at your high school or in your other activities (e.g., teaching piano lessons, helping to coach the volleyball team, taking a position on student council, or running the school Amnesty International club).

- Apply for, and keep track of, academic and other awards and accomplishments that you might include in your future medical-school application.

- Value all activities for their ability to teach you something—even activities that might not seem related to medicine. For example, working in the service sector can give you experience dealing with money, getting along with grumpy people, managing your time, and working in hot, busy, boring, stressful, or dirty environments.

University

Many of the strategies for high school students apply to university students as well, so please review the high school section. However, know that you will likely experience an increased academic workload in university, compared to high school. Plus, if you are not living at home, you may also be responsible for taking care of your own daily-living needs, such as grocery shopping, taking yourself to the doctor when you have strep throat, paying bills, and arranging to fix the squeaky fridge door. My students often refer to this as "adulting" (and comment on how tiring it is). In university, you may need to:

- Choose new activities, in a potentially new community or location, some connected to your university, some not.
- Decide how many activities you can balance with school and the other demands on your time.
- Start to assess and reflect on the patterns your activities have or will display: What picture of you do they create?
- Begin to track and write down roles, dates, locations, organizations, and verifiers.
- Add to an existing résumé with a view to applying to medical school.
- Reflect on your activities. Ask yourself: What did I learn? What did I contribute? Where do I have gaps? Can I or should I fill them before I apply? What am I most passionate about?
- Continue to track activities, awards, accomplishments, and verifiers.
- Consider potential referees for references, and set up meetings with them to discuss your career goals, experiences, and medical-school hopes.
- Access any medical-school application assistance available to you through your campus (e.g., career centre, residence advisors, academic advisors, professors).

Graduate school or after-undergraduate studies

If you are attending or have attended certain kinds of graduate school programs—for example, research programs—you may be required to submit a supplementary CV with your application. If you have graduated some time ago from any program, you may need to revive this type of information from a dated file. To complete this effectively, you may wish to:

- Connect with your supervisor, program leaders, or mentors who might be in a position to support your application to medical school.
- Stay somewhat diversified in your activities, even though you might not have summers off, and may be out of "school mode," with responsibilities such as teaching, marking, research, romantic or marital partners, and children.
- Assess your application for "gaps": think about what to start, what to keep doing, what to drop, and why.

- Start reconnecting with, or finding, people with whom you have worked or played in the past, so that you can build your verifier and reference list.
- Reflect on your activities. Ask yourself: What did I learn? What did I contribute? Where do I have gaps? Can I or should I fill them before I apply? What am I most passionate about?

Common mistakes and missed opportunities

My experience working with thousands of students applying to medical school over the past twenty years has helped me develop a list of common mistakes and missed opportunities in creating supplemental materials.

These include:

- spelling errors, typos, and grammatical errors
- listing every activity you have ever done, instead of choosing carefully those activities that best illustrate the contributions, skills, and qualities valued in medicine
- using labels that are not helpful or descriptive
- using descriptions that are vague and lack specificity
- failing to consider the big picture, so that the activities you include don't add up to a cohesive picture of a strong applicant
- including mostly structured activities, without considering informal activities

Writing strategies

I advise you to take deliberate steps to avoid the common pitfalls, and to craft a well-thought-out autobiographical sketch, CV, or résumé.

BRAINSTORM

Initially, you might want to simply brainstorm all your activities: roles, locations, organizations, and dates. Some students find it helpful to leave themselves voicemails or texts when they think of things during the day. For each medical school to which you apply, follow the instructions about start dates for recording your activities (e.g., some medical schools ask you to include activities starting at age sixteen, or starting with your undergraduate degree).

DESCRIBE

Maybe you're having trouble writing about what you did during an activity. Try telling a friend (or your voicemail) what you did. This process can help you record the major points, ensuring you can communicate the basic elements of the activity.

DETAIL

Detailing what you did in each activity is important. I suggest breaking this step into three parts.

First, think about yourself. (Everyone does this fairly well.) For example:

> "I worked with patients with disabilities for two years."

Next, think about yourself in relation to what medical schools state they are seeking in applicants.(Some students forget about this part.) For example:

> "I worked with a variety of patients with disabilities for two years and developed excellent compassion and patience."

Finally , describe your activities in ways that connect you to them, and to qualities sought by medical schools. (Most students don't do this well.) For example:

> "Working with patients with multiple sclerosis, muscular dystrophy, and Down syndrome developed my physical strength, compassion, and ability to communicate in diverse ways. I grew adept with daily bathing, feeding, and care routines, and gained exposure to assistive tools, including wheelchairs, Bliss boards, and basic American Sign Language."

Note that this example contains specific description as well as reflection on the activity—some insight into what you learned about yourself that could be valuable to a career in medicine.

I'm not saying this is easy, or that this is a "perfect" example. The character limit in some applications can make including detail a challenge. But, consider how you can make your writing more effective.

ORDER

If you are submitting a CV or résumé, decide on your section categories and list your activities in reverse chronological order (most recent to oldest) within each section, if not directed otherwise by the medical school.

If you are submitting an autobiographical sketch through OMSAS, the online system will do this for you.

PRIORITIZE AND RANK

Now, scrutinize your activities. Make sure you have included any activities identified as compulsory by the medical schools you are applying to. For other activities, ask yourself: Which were the easiest to write about? If they were easier to write about, this may be a clue that they were more meaningful to you, or that they helped you develop and grow in new ways. Also ask yourself: When did I see a problem and initiate a solution? Give these activities priority over activities where you were perhaps simply a "member." Pay attention to activities that feel significant, and distinguish them from activities that feel less significant.

EDIT, GET FEEDBACK, REWRITE

Because spelling and writing are essential parts of ensuring that readers can digest your autobiographical sketch, CV, or résumé with ease, it's important to use spell-check software—but don't rely on it solely. Here's a case in point: "My interest in medial school began when I helped care for my grandfather." *Medial* is a word, so spell-check software will not flag it as an error. But, you meant to type *medical*, didn't you?

It might not seem like a big deal to have a small error like this, but some readers might interpret these types of mistakes as a lack of attention to detail, or a lack of professionalism.

Have other people read your autobiographical sketch, CV, or résumé, and give you feedback. You can ask family, friends, advisors, or medical-school students, residents, and physicians. (Make sure, though, through all this process, that *you* are writing your supplemental materials: feedback should not become authorship.) Choose people you trust, who will help you and not crush your spirit: you need supportive and constructive feedback. Your best first reader might be a parent, but you may find value in more neutral readers (who don't already think you're wonderful) at some point before you submit.

Character limits

You may face character limits for each activity you include (e.g., autobiographical sketches submitted through OMSAS have character limits). This can pose challenges in providing enough description and detail to fully inform the reader. Use active language that is honest and vivid.

For example, instead of describing an activity like this:

"Helped patients with daily tasks" (32 characters)

You could describe it like this:

"Patient assistant" (17 characters)

This saves you 15 characters and is just as, if not more, clear. Think in terms of job titles and roles that accurately and honestly describe what you did (even if you didn't have an official job or volunteer title).

Unhelpful labels

Strive to be *descriptive* when you describe your activities. Look for ways to communicate quickly and succinctly, in case readers don't have time to get into the details.

Here are some examples of what I mean, based on an autobiographical sketch submitted through OMSAS. OMSAS examples are particularly important: the online OMSAS form for the autobiographical sketch allows you to click entries in the "description" column to add detail, but some Ontario medical schools skip that click when they read the form. They will only see the labels you use to summarize your activities.

Unhelpful labels: In my experience, many autobiographical sketch entries look something like this:

#	CAT	DATE RANGE	DESCRIPTION	GEOGRAPHIC LOCATION
1	E	2018/09–ongoing	Summer student	St. John's, NL
2	V	2018/09–2019/01	Volunteer	St. John's, NL

It's difficult, from the vague language in the "description" section, to get a good sense of what the student did.

Somewhat helpful labels: The following "description" section is slightly better, but still not as vivid as it could be.

#	CAT	DATE RANGE	DESCRIPTION	GEOGRAPHIC LOCATION
1	E	2018/09–ongoing	Summer student in lab	St. John's, NL
2	V	2018/09–2019/01	Hospital volunteer with patients	St. John's, NL

Can a reader picture fairly clearly what you did from these labels? Yes, in a general way, but many or most other candidates will also be describing work as a "summer student in lab" or "hospital volunteer with patients."

Plus, this wording wastes valuable characters, in my view. Your "summer student in lab" is repetitive because that entry already has a date with it (indicating summer). And you're obviously a student. So, only the "lab" part of this description is helpful. "Lab" is a pretty generic term, though, and doesn't help me remember or distinguish you from other sketches I'm reading.

Better labels: Let's try again.

#	CAT	DATE RANGE	DESCRIPTION	GEOGRAPHIC LOCATION
1	E	2018/09– ongoing	Research Asst, ovarian cancer	St. John's, NL
2	V	2018/09– 2019/01	Alzheimer Patient Activities Asst	St. John's, NL

Do you see how much more vivid these short descriptions are? They don't use lots of characters, but they help a reader "see" your activity more specifically. Strive for this type of writing for every activity in your sketch.

When you're crafting and editing your sketch, be sure to read your entries without clicking the "details" portion of the document: see whether each entry is descriptive enough, without that click, to be useful to a reader who doesn't know you and is evaluating your candidacy.

Similarly, when you're finishing a CV or résumé, consider whether you have created short, vivid headers, organizing terms, and role labels for each activity you include. These may be the only parts of your CV or résumé readers will retain.

Item order

In the OMSAS autobiographical sketch, you may enter items in any order. For example, you might start entering items from this year, because they are the easiest to remember and then save your document. Later, you might return and fill in a few items from high school, in a variety of categories. Provided you have included the requested dates for each item, OMSAS will reorder them in the way medical schools wish them to appear, before sending your application on.

If you are writing a CV or résumé, you need to order your activities yourself. The standard order is most recent to least recent, but check each medical school to which you apply for their particular instructions about CVs and résumés.

The "details" section of a sketch, CV, or résumé

Some medical schools give you the opportunity to include extra detail about your activities. The first thing to note is that not every medical school looks at the details during their review process.

It is crucial that your details—whether added to an autobiographical sketch, CV, or résumé—provide high-quality information to readers.

INSIDER INSIGHT

If you are applying to Ontario medical schools (through OMSAS), review carefully which schools examine details and ensure that your basic "description" information for each activity—the label you use to summarize what you did—is vivid enough for those who don't look at details.

For strategies on how to make your descriptions and details more effective, go back to the section in this chapter on writing strategies.

Note

1. "OMSAS—Autobiographical Sketch," Ontario Universities' Application Centre, accessed June 18, 2018, https://www.ouac.on.ca/guide/omsas-sketch/.

10

Personal essays and short answers

The evolution of written responses

Many students have come to me over the years groaning about all the writing they had to do for their medical-school applications. Most medical schools used to require an essay or responses to short-answer questions—some kind of writing that involved paragraphs—as part of their application process. At the University of Toronto, the essay word limit used to be 1,000 words. Some short-answer questions required candidates to respond in less than 700 characters (not words).

Maybe you feel like groaning about writing, too, and are relieved that most medical-school applications no longer ask for essays or short answers. Maybe not: maybe you think your writing skills might have boosted your application.

Essays and short answers took time and attention. The topics and questions were all just different enough, from one medical school to another, that applicants had to craft different sentences (or at least some different sentences) for each application. It was a lot of work for applicants. For my part as someone who used to screen medical-school applications, and had to read essays and short answers, it was a lot of work for me, too.

This is just one part of applying to medical school that has changed in the twenty years that I've been working with applicants.

If your parent or friend applied to medical school more than ten years ago, they can be a very helpful resource, but they probably didn't complete the application elements that you will today. That's not to say that their perspective isn't valuable, but their experience will not exactly fit what you will experience. I expect the same will be true for you, when you want to help guide some medical-school hopeful in the future.

How writing isn't going away

Some medical schools still request responses to short-answer questions (e.g., the University of Toronto), or reflections on your activities (e.g., McGill University). In my view, some schools have moved away from essays and short answers because they have found other application elements—including the CASPer system (covered in the next chapter)—as effective or more effective in screening candidates.

Each school seems to constantly refine and retool its application process, so—as with all the information in this resource—be sure to check with each medical school for its current application process in the year you will apply.

If you're applying to the University of Ottawa (and others) and going through the CASPer system, make no mistake about it: you'll still be writing. Some schools may also still include writing as part of their process, but it may occur in the context of a different element. For example, a school could make a writing station as part of a multiple mini-interview process.

> **INSIDER INSIGHT**
> If you haven't been engaged in much writing in recent years, or the language of your applications is not your first language, you may want to seek out opportunities at school or elsewhere to write persuasively and effectively, in preparation for applying to medical school.

Here are some general tips for writing, no matter where it occurs in your application process:

- Read the instructions carefully for each school.
- Strictly observe all character or word limits (note that a maximum length does not imply that you must use all those words or characters).
- Write well in advance of the due date (if possible) and worry

about containing your thoughts within the required length later, when editing.

- If permitted, have others read your writing and give feedback.

TIPS FOR HIGH SCHOOL AND EARLY UNIVERSITY
In high school and university, consider engaging in a writing-related activity, such as a writing-based course or club (e.g., the school events blog) to help keep your skills current.

What students do wrong with written responses: an example

Let's pretend you're a reader (like I was) for medical-school applications. You're reviewing multiple applications (let's say twenty-five) and every applicant has been asked to answer the same four short-answer questions. We'll look at the first question.

Q: Why do you want to be a doctor? (Please explain in less than 500 characters.)

Candidate 1 answers:

A: As I approach graduation and set my personal and professional goals, I have made a conscious decision to enter a field that would provide me with a sense of accomplishment and, at the same time, produce a positive impact on humankind. It became apparent to me that practising medicine would fulfill these objectives. In hindsight, my ever-growing commitment to medicine has been solidifying for years. My strong interest in social issues, education, and athletics seems particularly appropriate to this field and has prepared me well for such an important choice. (475 characters)

Candidate 2 answers:

A: I've been asked many times why I wish to become a doctor. Upon considerable reflection, the thought of having the skills to help others provides me with a tremendous feeling of satisfaction and offers the feeling that my life's efforts have been focused in a positive direction. Becoming a doctor is the culmination of a lifelong dream, and I am prepared to dedicate myself, as I have in the past, to achieving this goal. (347 characters)

You have read these two candidates' answers. Now, think about these questions: How do you tell the difference between these two candidates? Which candidate demonstrates informed choice? Which connects their own experiences to their answer? How do you assess whether the candidates give truthful answers? How would you grade their answers?

These two candidates have fallen victim to many of the most common weaknesses in short answers and essays. They:

- are so general that they could be anyone
- oversummarized their experiences so that they no longer have any distinctiveness or meaning
- don't connect their answer with a specific situation that is unique to them
- don't pick **one** experience that illuminates their answer
- removed anything that helps the reader remember them

Compare those answers to this answer:

A: It was a kazoo that first turned my thoughts to medicine. We were playing with neighbours and, as the eldest child, overseeing my siblings was my job. We were playing music: all of us banging on flowerpots, my sister belting out tunes on a kazoo. Suddenly, she choked and turned purple. I rushed over and gave an almighty "whack" on her back. She spit out a plastic piece from the kazoo. After my breathing calmed, I realized I was hooked on being able to save someone's life. But I realized I had lots to learn. Surely "whacking" wasn't an approved procedure? So, at age eleven, I began to dream of being a doctor. (500 characters)

This is not the "right" answer (that doesn't really exist), but it is a much more helpful answer—to the applicant's case and for the reader. While it doesn't completely cover all that might be needed to fully answer the question, it does a much better job than the previous examples, because:

- It is memorable (this might be filed "the kazoo person" in the reader's mind).
- It connects a specific example from the candidate's life to their reason for wanting to pursue medicine.
- It's vivid (you can almost see the child standing over the sibling).

- It sounds genuine (this kind of specificity can be hard to fabricate).
- It shows reflection ("I realized I had a lot to learn").

Strategies for written responses

Follow a consistent process

When you get a short-answer question:

- Underline or highlight key parts of the question.
- Make a list of the qualities or values that relate to the question and medicine.
- Choose **one** example from your life.
- Outline the steps, approach, or tactics that show the qualities or values in point form.
- Compose your answer.
- Go back and ensure you have answered all parts of the question.
- Edit for word length if you are over the limit.
- Have others read your answer for clarity, specificity, and meaning.

Cut to the chase

If you are used to writing long essays in high school or university, you have likely developed a fairly lengthy style of writing that includes introductions, hypotheses, evidence, and conclusions. This style of writing is generally too wordy for medical-school applications.

> **INSIDER INSIGHT**
>
> If you have a word limit for medical-school short answers or essays, you need to launch into the "evidence" part of your writing quickly. You don't have the space for long introductory paragraphs and repetition.

Many candidates (most I have worked with) start with statements that repeat the question (very unnecessary) or use a lot of words to restate the question (again, unnecessary). Here's an example.

Q: The Canadian health-care system faces many cost burdens today. Discuss two of the most difficult burdens, in your opinion, and how you might begin to solve them.

Typical answers start something like this:

A: This question asks me to consider the implications of cost on the current health-care system . . .

Or:

A: The current health-care system is very cumbersome and overloaded with many challenging costs to patients, caregivers, and practitioners . . .

If you are faced with a word or character limit, you don't have enough space to restate the question, in any way. Even if you do not have a limit, it's not a very compelling or wise use of the available space, which is your opportunity to stand out.

Use specific examples to tell your story

If you are required to complete short-answer questions or essays as part of your application process, you might begin by making some point-form notes. Let's work through an example.

Q: Describe a time when your active listening skills really paid off. What was the outcome? What might the outcome have been had you not actively listened?

A typical answer often looks like this:

A: Active listening is extremely important, especially when working with vulnerable people. Volunteering has taught me that many clues come

ASK YOURSELF
Does this response answer all parts of the question (or any of it)? Does it give evidence that helps a reader believe my answer?

from observing body language and maintaining good eye contact with people. As a volunteer at a retirement residence, I often found that listening helped me advocate for patients who wouldn't otherwise have spoken up about a problem they had. These patient experiences will be helpful for my future career as a doctor.

This answer is not "bad," but it misses some opportunities. It also doesn't get to the specificity that the question demands. It overgeneralizes about the character and experiences of the applicant. Hint: if you are using words such as *often* and *these experiences*, you might be oversummarizing.

USING SPECIFIC EXAMPLES, STEP BY STEP

Let's work through the question about active listening together.

First, you might want to separate the parts of the question to ensure that you don't neglect to answer something.

The question has three parts:

1. Describe a time when your active listening skills really paid off.
2. What was the outcome?
3. What might the outcome have been had you not actively listened?

Now, answer each part separately, so you can be sure that your answer is complete.

Q Part 1. Describe a time when your active listening skills really paid off.

Think about this. When you have used active listening skills? You might first think:

> My roommate was having some issues last year and I helped her by using active listening skills.

This is a good start—but don't write this in your application and leave it. You're still oversummarizing at this point. Think about how to make your answer more specific and vivid.

> Last year, my roommate started telling me that she was "just not hungry" and began refusing invitations to go out with our friends.

Much better! You have isolated a particular incident or set of incidents to answer the question. Now, you need to help the reader understand the situation.

> While she didn't share much info, it was clear that she was struggling, so I just listened to her and eventually suggested counselling.

This is helpful because it describes something specific that happened and that you **took action on**.

Now, let's go to the next parts of the question.

Q Part 2. What was the outcome?

> She began to get treatment for an eating disorder and was feeling much better.

Q Part 3. What might the outcome have been had you not actively listened?

She told me later that she had been contemplating suicide, but because of my nonjudgemental listening, she felt better enough to realize that she needed help and she began to get counselling.

Okay, now let's put it all together and edit it, so that it fits within the word limit.

Q (all parts): Describe a time when your active listening skills really paid off. What was the outcome? What might the outcome have been had you not actively listened?

A: Last year, my roommate started telling me that she was "just not hungry" and began refusing invitations to go out with our friends. While she didn't share much info, it was clear that she was struggling, so I just listened to her and eventually suggested counselling. She told me later that she had been contemplating suicide, but because of my nonjudgemental, active listening, she began to get treatment for an eating disorder and was feeling more positive.

This example is not meant to serve as a "perfect" specimen, but rather to help you understand what components can make your answers more effective and memorable.

General outline of a personal statement

I am not aware of medical schools that currently require a full personal statement or essay, unless you are applying outside Canada. However, if you are applying under a special category, you may be asked to submit a supplementary piece of writing: a letter, a personal statement, or a statement of intent.

Follow the instructions given, but if you are simply asked to submit "a statement" or letter, you might consider addressing some or all of the following:

- a statement about why you want to pursue medicine
- evidence that you are a good risk for medical school and have related experience
- information related to the special category you are applying under

- how completing an MD dovetails with your next steps or goals
- why you are applying to this institution and location
- conclusion

All the same guidelines for short-answer questions apply to personal statements and letters. Be wary of the extra space you may have: avoid filling it with words that aren't on target for your cause.

11

Computer-based Assessment for Sampling Personal Characteristics

Test basics

CASPer is an online assessment of your interpersonal and decision-making skills. Medical schools that use CASPer generally require the test before they offer candidates interviews (often in November), and your score often determines whether you are invited for an interview.

CASPer consists of ten to twelve video-based or written scenarios. The test is ninety minutes (generally sixty-five minutes of test with an optional break). You need to complete CASPer in one sitting (i.e., you can't save and go back later).

Students often report to me that, of all the elements of the application process (except for interviews), CASPer makes them the most apprehensive. If you have family members who applied to medical school in the past, they probably did not have CASPer as part of their application process. Not every medical school uses it, but, with every passing year, it seems that more and more schools are incorporating it into their process. In time, it may become a standard element of medical-school applications.

In Canada, the following medical schools, so far, have opted for CASPer: Dalhousie University, McMaster University, McGill University, the University of Alberta, and the University of Ottawa. CASPer may be a requirement in other Canadian health-sciences programs, too (e.g., dentistry, physical therapy, optometry, and occupational therapy). A few American and Caribbean medical schools also use it.

Cost

In Canada, the fee is currently $40 to take the test plus a $10 distribution fee for each school to which you are sending the results (plus any applicable taxes).

Where and how you take CASPer

The test is online, so you can take it from a computer and location of your choosing. There are technical requirements you need to meet to run the test (e.g., broadband; secure, stable Internet; webcam). Be sure to test your Internet connection before you book and pay for your CASPer date. As a rural resident, I can tell you that my slow and patchy "country Internet" would not work for taking CASPer.

Using a tablet is **not** recommended by the testing site.

You need to register for the test. To register, you need government-issued photo ID (e.g., driver's license, passport). You also need your school application ID number, which allows you to sign in and book a test date and time. Note that each school may have specific deadlines for accepting your CASPer results—be sure that you are choosing test dates that comply with their requirements.

Visit the CASPer website for more information about dates, procedures, and more (use *takecasper* as the search term in your browser).

Where CASPer fits in the application process

Currently, medical schools seem to use CASPer scores as a way to assess which candidates are most suitable for interviews. Some schools may use it in lieu of interviews, but I am not aware of any Canadian programs that do this.

Therefore, pay attention to any minimum CASPer score the schools you are applying to require.

Accommodations

If you require accommodations for this assessment, you must submit a formal request and supporting documentation well in advance of your test. Check the CASPer website for specific guidelines about what is required, and when, so you won't have to add this to your stress on test day.

How to prepare for CASPer

Students have reported to me that the following strategies—although basic and obvious in some ways—helped them with their CASPer performance. If you're still in high school or early university when starting these strategies, you have more than the usual time to develop skills that will help you with CASPer, if and when you decide to take it in the future.

Practise typing and try to increase your speed. This might sound silly, but don't assume you have this skill. Many students text with ease, but they can't type very quickly on a conventional keyboard. Adept keyboard typing can help you answer CASPer questions more efficiently in the time provided.

Here are some ideas to help you increase your keyboarding speed in a fairly short time. First (get ready for a really old-fashioned idea), *sit at a full keyboard* (not in a reclined position, not with a tablet or phone), and then:

- Use your social media this way, for a few weeks.
- Use online programs that help you practise touch-typing.
- Type the words to your favourite songs as you listen to them.
- Try to type every word a teacher or professor says during class.
- Type while you listen to podcasts: try to keep up with the dialogue.
- Retype news articles or passages from books.

The occasional typo or spelling mistake should not affect your CASPer score, but you want to ensure that your answers make sense and are legible.

Think about the kinds of interpersonal and decision-making skills a medical student or doctor would need, since CASPer assesses interpersonal and decision-making skills. Some examples of these skills include:

- making a connection with a stranger
- demonstrating kindness, empathy, compassion
- making difficult decisions when there's no "right" answer
- managing conflict
- balancing competing rights among individuals
- making an unpopular decision

- calming someone down or defusing a situation
- being firm even when challenged

EXERCISE: CHART YOUR SKILLS FOR CASPer
In a column, write down the skills from the list I made (add other skills—my list is not a complete list). After each skill, write down a specific example from your life that demonstrates you employing the skill. Then, describe each example using the CAR method (context, action, results). For example, the following might illustrate the skill of defusing a situation:

    Context: "Last Thursday at the basketball game . . . "
    Action: "First, I decided to . . . "
    Result: "In the end, we all calmed down and I realized . . . "

Hanging your answer on this structure can help you describe your experience with useful detail and in a logical way.

You may also find it helpful to think of examples from your life when you **did not** usefully employ a skill. Then, ask yourself (and write down in your chart), What steps could I have taken? What could I have said or done? Who could I have involved? Where could I have found more help? (Remember, in real life, you don't need to work alone.)

Finally, think about skills in terms of situations you have not experienced. For example, what about defusing a situation in an emergency department, where a family member is upset at an injured patient for driving drunk? What about a patient who becomes angry because you refuse to refill their opioid prescription?

Read articles and books about ethics, including *Doing Right: A Practical Guide to Ethics for Medical Trainees and Physicians* by Philip Hebert (Oxford University Press, 2014) to help you get a sense of how to deal with medical ethics and issues that may have more than one answer.

Do some interview preparation, because the questions and scenarios on CASPer seem to echo many typical medical-school interview questions.

Choose a time and date when you will be at your best. Not a morning person? Schedule your test later in the day.

Do a practice run. Test your equipment and any sample questions you can get in advance of the test (e.g., practice scenarios).

Get enough sleep and rest before your CASPer date. This tends to help with concentration and critical thinking in most people.

Gather anything that might help you during the test—your lucky charm, pad and paper, notes you've made in preparation, and so on. Think carefully about whether these will actually help you or end up as distractions, or take up valuable time or attention during the test.

Clear your space of distractions. Turn off your phone, tell your family or housemates that you will need quiet for ninety minutes, or schedule your test when no one will be home. Be sure you're not running (and no one else is running) bandwidth-hogging programs that will affect how CASPer works.

Take a deep breath, and, using all your preparation, **begin.**

Sample questions

The CASPer website has sample video scenarios with questions (use *takecasper* as the search term in your browser).

A scenario

Let's try working through an example together (an example I have made up). This, of course, will be a written scenario.

Your role in this scenario: friend.

Scenario: Your friend has had four seizures in the last few weeks and has recently been diagnosed with epilepsy. He has just started taking medication, but the seizures have not stopped yet. His doctor has told your friend that he is not safe to drive, and that the doctor's office has notified the Ministry of Transportation to remove your friend's license because it is against the law to drive until seizures are managed for at least one year.

You see your friend driving to hockey practice and when you call him on it, he gets angry. He says that he can tell when he's going to have a seizure and he is perfectly safe on the road. He says that you're "not a doctor" and to mind your own business.

QUESTIONS:

1. What do you say to your friend?
2. If your friend doesn't agree to stop driving, how would you handle it?

In addition to the time limit for the test as a whole, particular scenarios may have particular time limits. If you have a time limit for your response to this scenario, you might want to quickly decide approximately how much of the time you allot to question 1, question 2, and reviewing and editing.

Next, consider the possible issues involved in the scenario. For example:

- Your friend has a new and possibly frightening diagnosis.
- He is putting himself and others in danger by continuing to drive.
- He is breaking the law.
- He says he thinks he has warnings of his seizures, but he may be wrong, or he may not be telling the truth.

Finally, ask yourself, Who are the people affected by the situation in the scenario? In this case, the situation affects:

- your friend
- the people who might be put at risk because of his actions

Now, look at the questions. You want to ensure that you answer everything.

Q 1: What do you say to your friend?

A: My friend has a new and possibly frightening diagnosis of epilepsy. First, I would try to show him that I care by expressing concern about him and asking him how he is doing with this new situation. I want him to feel that I understand some of what he is going through and am there to be a friend to him. I would listen to him and then tell him that I understand why he wants to drive, but I'm concerned for his safety. I want to help him come to a good solution about how to get around while he waits to get his seizures under control.

Or:

A: I'm really sorry that you've been going through this. It must be very difficult to deal with something like seizures and a diagnosis of epilepsy. How are you feeling about all this? Is there anything I can do to help you? I'm also happy to just listen, if you need to talk. (I'd listen for a while). I'm sorry that I made you feel bad about driving, but I was concerned. I really care about you and don't want anything to happen to you. Since this is new, I'm not sure you really would know if a seizure was coming on, in time. I can't imagine losing my license. That must be really difficult! What if I came to pick you up for hockey practice instead? We could also talk about ideas for how you could get around until you're feeling better and you get your driver's license back.

Neither of these approaches to question 1 is necessarily a "perfect answer." I include them so that you have a chance to think like a reviewer. Candidates might choose to answer someone hypothetically or actually address their remarks as if they're talking directly to the person involved in the question. Either method could be a possible approach for your answer. Unless instructed otherwise, choose the writing voice that works best for your style and the question.

Now you must answer the second question.

Q 2: If your friend doesn't agree to stop driving, how would you handle it?

A: It's against the law to drive while seizures are not controlled, so I would encourage him to promise not to drive. I would help him strategize about ways to get around until he gets his seizures under control. I'd offer to go with him to support groups where he could meet others who are struggling with seizures and loss of license. I'd offer to drive him places, if it would help. I'd encourage him to contact his doctor, if he has questions about anything, including driving. If he still wouldn't stop, I would tell him that I would have to notify his parent and/or physician, because I am really concerned about his safety and the safety of others.

Or:

A: You told me that your doctor said you can't drive until the seizures are under control and the Ministry of Transportation gives you permission again. I don't want to see

---

ASK YOURSELF

Did I consider multiple sides of an issue or factors in a decision?

Did I follow rules or break them? Have I defended my choice?

Do I know when something should be reported? (Note that scenarios will inform you of relevant laws. You will be expected to know what do to with that information, and with information that has moral or ethical importance.)

Can I see things from a unique or different perspective that hasn't been shown or described in the scenario?

you get in trouble or arrested for driving without a license. I also don't want you to get hurt or have to deal with inadvertently hurting someone else, if you have an accident because of a seizure. I care about you, and if you won't stop driving on your own, I'm afraid I have to tell someone. I really wish we could do this together, but if you won't, I will have to tell your parents or your doctor that you are still driving. I know you might be angry with me, but it's important that you don't drive right now. I want to help you get better in any way I can, so that you can drive again as soon as possible. I am your friend and I'm on your side, but I hope you understand that I can't support your decision to drive right now.

Give yourself time during the test to review your answer.

Other types of questions

CASPer may also ask questions that require you to cite specific examples from your own experience.

For example: **Tell us about a time when you had to act as the leader in a situation. What was your approach? What did you find difficult?**

As with anything you write for medical-school applications—an autobiographical sketch, responses to short-answer questions—it's important to be vivid and specific to **your** experience. The question says, "Tell me about a time . . . "—so, you need to think of a specific incident to write about. Preparing your list of experiences, as I recommended in the exercise in this chapter, will help you immensely with these questions. You could also have a look at chapter 9 on writing an autobiographical sketch, CV, or résumé for more ideas about how to be as vivid as possible.

There are many websites with hundreds of sample ethical and situational questions for medical-school interviews. They are a great way to practise strategies and writing in advance of your CASPer.

12

References

Your transcripts and MCAT scores look amazing, and your supplemental materials are excellent—but what do other people say about you? Does what they say support the rest of your application? Do they raise any red flags?

Most medical schools ask applicants to supply references—comments from referees. The role of a referee is to give an "outside" perspective on your qualities, character, and capabilities.

References can be challenging, because they are a part of the application process that you don't really control. This chapter outlines strategies to help you maximize the chances that your referees provide strong, positive comments on your behalf.

The rules around referees

Referees are people who can attest to your personal qualities, character, academic capabilities, potential, and any special circumstances you've faced. Consider carefully any guidelines from the medical schools to which you are applying: What do they say referees should assess? What academic and nonacademic priorities does their website talk about? Choose your referees accordingly.

Ontario

In Ontario, the process of submitting references, as with other application elements, is centralized (through OMSAS). You need three references, and those three references go to every medical school in Ontario to which you apply. This means you won't be asking someone to be a referee for your application to the Northern Ontario School of Medicine, and someone else to be a referee for the University of Ottawa. OMSAS ensures only three references will be assessed across all Ontario medical schools, even if you submit more. In addition, at least one of your referees should supply a non-academic or character reference.

Through OMSAS, each referee completes a confidential reference form and submits it directly to the online system. The form, when I have acted as a referee, asks for comments

> **INSIDER INSIGHT**
> You have three opportunities to ensure that, taken together, your references represent you in a well-rounded way.

on specific skills or qualities (e.g., communication skills), and the response is more or less like writing a letter. As an applicant using OMSAS, you will be electronically sending instructions and the form to each of your referees, after you have created your account. You will therefore need each referee's preferred email address.

Outside Ontario

In other provinces, each medical school has its own reference requirements and submission instructions. You could try to recruit different referees for each school to which you apply (e.g., you might ask someone from British Columbia to be your referee only for your application to the University of British Columbia medical school). However, this won't be practical for most applicants, so don't worry if it isn't practical for you.

You will likely not see what referees write about you, because referees are generally asked to submit their comments directly to the medical schools to which you apply. Some referees break this rule and show you their comments (I've even had students say referees have asked them to write letters of reference themselves and just bring them back for signing), but most often you won't know what they say. Because of this, it's important to choose people whom you think really support you and will take the time to write you a good reference.

Each referee may not be able to speak about every quality that medical schools have requested, but do ensure that the sum total of your reference letters covers all the requested characteristics.

How to choose referees

Bearing in mind any instructions from the medical schools to which you are applying, choose referees who, alone or in combination, will do the best job for you. That is, choose people whose comments will support, solidify, or extend the information a reviewer will have already seen in your application. Given that medical-school applicants are assessed on a combination of academic and other characteristics, you should also consider how referees will help you present a combination of attributes.

Typical referee categories

Most students find the following categories helpful in sorting through possible referees.

- **Academic referees:** These are teachers or professors who have evaluated you (i.e., taught you a class and marked you). Sometimes a teaching assistant for a university course knows you better than the professor of the course. In this case, the professor should still be the referee, but ask for the teaching assistant to help the professor write the reference.
- **Referees from employment or volunteer work:** These are people who have supervised your work—whether you were paid or not.
- **Character referees:** These are people who have known you in some depth and are perhaps bound by the ethical code of a professional association (which adds to their reliability as commentators). Many students use family doctors, coaches, police officers, judges, or business owners they know. Bear in mind that all references should be objective—**not** family members, peers, or friends of your family.

Many students, especially in university, are supervised by other students. I would not use another student as a medical-school referee. Students who have supervised you, however, might provide examples of your skills or characteristics to a responsible teacher, professor, or staff person who is writing a reference for you.

When and how to start looking for referees

START AS SOON AS POSSIBLE
Even if you're in high school or early university, think about who might write you a strong, positive reference.

Many medical-school applicants use a high school principal or teacher, or a university professor, as one of their referees. This is not essential, but it makes sense from the point of view that students spend a lot of time with educators. However, beware of seeking all your referees among people who knew you best several years ago. Other popular options for referees include coaches, music teachers, youth group leaders, family doctors, and volunteer or work supervisors.

ASK YOURSELF

Who really thinks I am amazing?

Who gives me the best grades?

Who asks me about my future and seems to have high hopes for my prospects?

Who has helped me develop, or been a mentor to me?

Who has been great to work or volunteer with?

Who has offered to be a referee for me?

When choosing referees, consider:

- how well they know you (ideally, they have in-depth knowledge of you)
- how long have they known you (sometimes longer is better, but not always—consider the depth of knowledge)
- how enthusiastic about you and supportive of you they are
- whether they seem to have time to be a good referee
- whether you have any sense of their writing style (too curt might sound negative, too exuberant might lack credibility)
- who is in the best position to write about you in detail and with examples

Keep track of potential referees as you go along. Stay in touch from time to time, so you know where to find them, when the time comes.

CULTIVATE RELATIONSHIPS

Students in high school or university, especially in large classes, might not make the effort to get to know a teacher or professor. Some students feel nervous with an employer or supervisor, and don't get to know them. Remember: it's very normal to ask an instructor,

TIPS FOR HIGH SCHOOL AND EARLY UNIVERSITY

There is nothing wrong with cultivating and maintaining relationships that could provide you with referees.

employer, or supervisor for a reference. Also remember: it's a lot easier for them to write insightful comments about you when you are more than just a grade in their class or someone who showed up for every shift.

Ask questions, visit them during office hours, write thank-you notes at graduation, book an appointment to see them to discuss your ideas and future plans. Let them know you're thinking about medical school—and possible referees in the future. If you're graduating, make an effort to stay in touch with people you'd like to have as referees.

How to request a reference

Provide key details when you ask

The process of requesting a reference can be as informal or formal as you like, but I recommend erring on the side of more formal. (It makes a good impression.) You can email, text, or ask someone verbally to be a reference for you. When you do so, be sure to remind them of these details:

- your full name and contact information
- how they know you
- that you are applying to medical school
- that you would really appreciate them providing you a reference (a later section in this chapter covers how to ask)
- what's involved: the documents they have to submit, the deadlines you need them to meet

Make an appointment

Strong, positive reference letters provide details that describe you doing great things. They help support your application. You can imagine what a typical reference letter for a medical-school hopeful might say: "This candidate is amazing. Best student I've ever worked with. I highly recommend them to your medical school."

INSIDER INSIGHT

While it's not bad to be an amazing student and the best student someone has ever worked with, it's also probably not very different from what all the other referees are saying about other students.

A strong, positive reference—just like the autobiographical sketch, CV, or résumé you prepare yourself—needs to be vivid and specific. There are ways to (tactfully) help each of your referees achieve this. An easy way is to make an appointment with them to discuss the reference and your goals. This can help each referee catch up on your recent activities and understand more about the things you do outside their interactions with you. In this appointment, you can:

- Help them understand more about you, in other contexts (e.g., "Here's my résumé, in case you would like to see what else I'm involved with. I'd be happy to tell you about these activities").

- Remind them, gently, about things you've done in their sphere, accomplishments you've had, and obstacles you've overcome (e.g., "Remember that really intense basketball game where the opposing team fouled me and I sprained my ankle? Wow, I was happy I was able to get back on the team later that season").

- Ask them if they have any questions about what they have been asked to submit (and offer to find out the answer, if you don't know it).

- Ask if there is anything you can do to help them submit comments on your behalf (e.g., supply stamped, addressed envelopes, or send a reminder a week before the due date).

Ask, but with an "out"

I know it can be nerve-wracking to ask for a reference (or three), but don't worry. It's very normal to request a reference from a teacher, professor, employer, volunteer supervisor, coach, and others. Many students are nervous about appearing to "use" people, but for people in these roles, it's a regular occurrence to be asked to offer support in this way. In fact, it can be a wonderful way for people to feel like they're really helping you. And, most people like to help.

However, when you ask someone to act as your referee, I suggest you use this sentence: "Do you feel you know me well enough to provide a strong, positive reference for medical school for me?"

This gives your referees an "out." Maybe they feel they don't know you well enough, or maybe they feel they don't have enough to say to support your application, or maybe they don't really like you (!).

If this is the case, they can simply say, "Actually, I'm not sure I know you well enough. How about asking so-and-so for a reference?" It's a less awkward way for them to say no.

The second part of my suggested sentence is important to note, too. You want to ask specifically if they can write a **strong, positive** reference.

INSIDER INSIGHT

Although it can be disappointing when someone turns you down as a referee, it's better to be turned down than to include someone who may not submit a strong, positive reference.

Think about how enthusiastic all the other references for all the other medical-school applicants will be, when medical schools are reading them. You want yours to stand up to that level.

What makes a strong, positive reference?

In my opinion, a strong reference does your work for you: it supports your application, it confirms what those reviewing your application are already reading about you, and it may expand on some aspects of your application or provide useful new information about you. It doesn't need to be from a famous person. It just needs to be from someone who really thinks **you** are amazing, special, brilliant, hardworking, full of potential—and who can communicate that in writing.

When you specifically use the words *strong* and *positive* in asking for a reference, you help remind the potential referee that they are committing to something specific, if they say yes. You don't need "just a letter." You need something that will really enhance your application. If they feel they can't do this, for whatever reason, it's better for them to turn you down so you can ask someone else.

Students often ask me, "Should I choose the 'big name' over someone who knows me better?" Together, we strategize about the best combination of referees for their situation.

Some students choose a "bigger name" (e.g., a well-known scientist) as one referee, who perhaps knows them but not as well as someone else. They back this up with two very strong recommendations from people who really know them well. It's their decision—and yours.

INSIDER INSIGHT

I believe that it's always best to have strong recommendations from people who know you really well.

Avoid repetition in your references, if you can. For example, choosing three academic referees, who will only comment on this aspect of you, may not help medical schools see the full picture of your attributes. Likewise, choosing three character references might not give a full picture of your ability to learn or your drive for academic excellence.

Special circumstances

Referees are in a great position to help support your application and, in some cases, this means they can talk about something that's hard to explain in other ways. For example, I had a student who had battled cancer while in her undergraduate degree (you met her in chapter 7). She asked her referees to comment on her academic progress through this diagnosis and treatment. I believe one of her physicians acted as a referee for her, commenting on her fit with medicine in terms of her personality and as a cancer survivor.

Another student I know had a difficult time when his (mostly estranged) father unexpectedly died during his first year of university. This led to some mental health struggles for him: he mourned and felt conflicted for some time afterward. His academic transcript showed some of that struggle, but his references gave his application a place to describe what had happened. His referees helped those who reviewed his application understand how he successfully navigated that tragedy and its aftermath.

Another student had helped his mother with her mental health, through crisis after crisis, while in high school and university. She ultimately and tragically took her own life. His references attested to the strength of character he had demonstrated in the face of these challenges, and how determined he was to make positive changes for others someday, as a physician.

Cautions

While you only have so much control over your referees, I have seen a few things to avoid, if you can.

- **Avoid using a referee who does not speak the language of your application well.** Assess your referee's writing skills in the language of your application. I have had students ask about using a family doctor living in their family's home country as a referee. My question is always, How well does this potential referee write in English (or French)? A referee's lack of language skills may not be held against you, as the applicant, but it may make it difficult for reviewers to understand the referee's comments, and this can compromise your application.

- **Give your referees enough time to complete the task.** Help your referees clearly understand the deadlines they need to meet, and give them enough time to complete their task well. Most people need at least a few weeks in advance of the deadline. Make sure you ask about, and navigate around, your referees' vacation and other plans. If you are including professors as referees, watch out for sabbaticals (academic leave).

- **Avoid pestering your referees.** You are probably nervous. I understand that it can be very difficult to check your application status and see that someone hasn't submitted their comments. It's frustrating and nerve-wracking when an essential part of your application is not complete. It's okay to politely check if a referee is having any issues with submission and remind them of the deadline. You may also want to ask if there is anything they need from you. A couple of times is okay. However, at some point, you have to trust them to do what they have agreed to do. Pestering them constantly won't inspire them to think kindly of you.

- **Don't assume referees will send a good letter without any input from you.** Many applicants assume referees know how to write a helpful letter. In fact, they often don't. In the case of academic referees (teachers and professors), they may have more of a sense, but it can still be helpful to provide the information I suggest in this chapter. This is especially true for referees who do not work in education: they may never have written a reference for medical school before. This chapter has suggestions for ways to help them help you.

13

Interviews

The most-nervous people I have ever seen are students arriving for their medical-school interviews. As a group, these students are extremely talented, bright, and accomplished. Yet, interview day can bring out the shakes in the most confident of them. And no wonder: it feels like a major life crossroads—an opportunity that could make or break the rest of your life.

This chapter outlines strategies to help you succeed and put your best self forward during interviews. This involves thinking about your personal challenges with regard to interviews, and working on ways to overcome them. Practice, up to a point, can also help.

INSIDER INSIGHT
If you get invited to an interview, take some time to congratulate yourself. In this highly competitive process, getting an interview is a **big deal**. In most cases, it means you have made it through the first gauntlet of the application-review process and are among the much smaller group of applicants that schools want to meet in person.

One of my biggest sorrows, as a former medical-school interviewer, was knowing that the many qualified candidates, who had arrived at this stage, could not all be offered spots. If you get to the interview stage but don't get an offer, take heart: you are likely among the most promising candidates and I would encourage you to apply again in the future, if it makes sense for you.

How interviews work

Across the country, interviews tend to take place between January and March. Some schools interview in December, when students are home for the holiday break. If you are invited for an interview, a school might give you a schedule for the day, and let you know the interview

INSIDER INSIGHT

If you have a choice about when to conduct your interview, choose a date and time of day when you are at your best. I recommend this because, in most cases, your energy will help interviewers connect with and remember you.

format they have chosen. Often, schools simply notify you of your interview date and time without further details.

Accommodations

As with other parts of the application process, if you require accommodations for your interview, you need to notify the medical school well in advance of your interview dates so that they can arrange for your needs.

Types of questions in interviews

Medical-school interviews can engage any question among thousands of possibilities. This section explores some broad categories typical of many questions.

General or personal questions

This type of question may stem from reading your file, either before the interview or during it, or it may simply be a question that every candidate is asked. Examples of this type of question include:

Tell us about yourself.

Why do you want to be a doctor?

Why should we choose you over someone else?

What do you most want us to know about you?

Why did you choose your current degree?

Why do you want to get into medical school now, instead of finishing your degree?

You have a lot of social justice (or some other) experience: why not go into counselling instead?

STRATEGIES FOR GENERAL OR PERSONAL QUESTIONS

Review your autobiographical sketch, CV, or résumé thoroughly. Think about why you did what you did and what you learned from each activity (even older ones).

Make point-form notes about the reasoning behind your choice of medicine and the experiences that connect you to it. Be specific: "I love science and want to help people" will likely sound like every other candidate.

ASK YOURSELF

What experiences taught me that I love science?

How did I realize I loved helping people?

What other fields have I explored and what are they missing?

Behavioural questions

Behavioural questions ask you to describe an example from the past that helps interviewers predict your future behaviour. Often, these questions are based on specific qualities that medical schools are seeking. Examples of this type of question include:

Tell me about a time you had to give someone bad news.

Tell me about a time when you did a great job as a leader.

Tell us about a time when you tried to be a good team player, but it didn't go well.

Tell us about a time you failed.

Tell us about a time when you had to communicate with someone whose first language wasn't the same as yours. What were the challenges? How did you succeed?

STRATEGIES FOR BEHAVIOURAL QUESTIONS

Make a list of key attributes medical schools say they look for. Write point-form examples that demonstrate you engaging each attribute. (For a structured and logical answer, review the CAR method in chapter 11.) Then:

- Practise telling the point-form examples as stories, out loud.
- Tell the stories to your voicemail, so you can listen to yourself speak.
- Tell the stories to other people and ask for feedback.

Ethics questions

The practice of medicine is full of ethical dilemmas. Interviewers do not expect you to have the facility of a physician with these dilemmas, but your response to dilemmas helps them glean information about your potential. Often, questions about ethics have no absolute right or wrong answers. An appropriate answer may lie in examining different sides of an argument and presenting your case. Examples of this type of question include:

Do you think heroin addicts should be given free methadone treatments when cancer patients must pay for their medicines?

Should the hunting and fishing rights of Indigenous Peoples be curtailed with seasons and quotas?

Discuss the pros and cons of socialized medicine.

Should people with certain self-imposed health conditions (e.g., smoking-related lung cancer, weight-related diabetes, alcohol-related liver disease) pay for hospital visits?

Should parents who don't believe in blood transfusions be allowed to deny their infant child the right to a life-saving transfusion?

STRATEGIES FOR ETHICS QUESTIONS

Read *Doing Right: A Practical Guide to Ethics for Medical Trainees and Physicians* by Philip Hebert (Oxford University Press, 2014) for examples of dilemmas physicians face and how they handle them.

Think about your own belief systems and how you can show consideration for opposite viewpoints.

Consider the balance between logic and humanity, and cost and compassion.

Break down issues into smaller pieces or "buckets." Start by talking about those buckets, and then "dump the buckets" to expand on each issue.

Think about how you would defend your beliefs, if challenged.

Situational questions

Situational questions usually involve reading a scenario or listening to a scenario posed by interviewers. In some cases, they might involve role-playing.

Examples of this type of question include:

> You see someone cheating during a major exam. What, if anything, would you do at the time or after?
>
> You are asked by your underage coworker to buy a few beers for her and her friends. She says everyone plans to hang out in her basement and no one will be driving anywhere. She says she thinks this is safer than going out to a field party in the woods. How would you respond? Would you buy her the beer?
>
> Your grandmother tells you that she won't get the flu vaccine this year because it "doesn't work." She volunteers at a day care and says that her immune system is "bullet proof," especially because she also takes vitamin D. Several of the infants in her day care are not old enough to be vaccinated. How would you respond?
>
> You have been accused of stealing lab supplies from the summer research institute you work in. You have not stolen anything, but you have seen a coworker putting things in her knapsack several times. Walk in and deal with this situation.

INSIDER INSIGHT

Reviewers may be interested to see how you respond to difficult scenarios, how you communicate, how you work logically through a situation, and whether you can defuse tension, rather than letting tension fluster you.

There may be follow-up questions, after your initial response. The follow-up questions might be deliberately provocative: no matter how you first answered, the interviewers may take the opposite position, to see how you respond. Sometimes, you might even face a quite aggressive response (e.g., "That's a **really** stupid idea. Why on earth would you do that?"). It's normal to feel quite flustered, faced with this behaviour, but try to stay calm. Mature people will acknowledge other people's viewpoints and feelings, and are able to stay on point or politely disagree.

STRATEGIES FOR SITUATIONAL QUESTIONS

You can use the same strategies to prepare for situational questions as for ethics questions:

- Think about your own belief systems and how you can show consideration for opposite viewpoints.
- Consider the balance between logic and humanity, and cost and compassion.

- Break down issues into smaller pieces or "buckets." Start by talking about those buckets, and then "dump the buckets" to expand on each issue.
- Think about how you would defend your beliefs, if challenged.

When faced with a situational question, you might also think about whether you have experienced something similar, and mention briefly how that experience informed the actions and decisions in your response.

Questions about current events, opinions, and decisions

As a former medical-school interviewer and as a prospective patient, I always hope that any medical school candidate cares about what's happening in the world. Examples of these types of questions include:

Who is the current provincial health minister? Federal health minister?

Tell us about three nonheadline issues you have been following.

How would you solve the Crimean crisis?

What do you think is the biggest health issue facing patients in our region?

Tell us what you know about issues currently facing oil sands development in Alberta.

Tell me what you know about the change in euthanasia laws in Canada.

As you can see, this type of question can be impossible to predict and can cover—quite literally—a world of material. Staying up to date with what's happening in your region, in Canada, and in the world is really important.

STRATEGIES FOR CURRENT EVENTS QUESTIONS

Your life may be busy: it can be easy to get cocooned in your bubble of activities and studies. I work with many medical-school hopefuls. I encourage all of them, and you, to:

- Follow your local, regional, and broader news.
- Pay attention to health topics.
- Think about the locations of the medical schools to which

you are applying, and pay attention to issues of importance in those locations.

- Know what you know. It's nearly impossible to follow or know everything about the world. It might help to explain your lack of knowledge in a specific area if you can say (at least), "I tend to follow humanitarian and human rights (or some other) issues, and I know only a little about what you've asked me, but here is what I know."

- Don't guess. Always let interviewers know if you are making an educated guess. It's better to say the little you know about an issue than to fabricate something.

Off-the-wall questions

I used to interview with someone (when we were hiring physicians) who loved asking off-the-wall questions. He felt that it helped him get at the "real" candidate—one that wasn't so rehearsed and coached. I feel that these types of questions can be unfair to people who like to pause and think. Nevertheless, you may encounter some of these during your interviews. Examples of this type of question include:

If you could be any kitchen appliance, what would you be?

Who is your favourite person, living or dead?

What book is on your bedside table right now?

What's your favourite day of the week?

Teach me something in the next five minutes.

Give me a word for each letter of your first name.

Do the best you can when faced with these questions, and remember that one less-than-stellar answer does not usually sink your whole interview.

STRATEGIES FOR OFF-THE-WALL QUESTIONS

Take time to think. You are **always** allowed time to think. It can feel awkward to pause and think, but it may help you with these and other types of questions. I would also recommend letting interviewers know that you are going to think (e.g., "I need to think about that for a moment"), as opposed to simply going quiet with no explanation.

Be careful with humour. It can be tempting to be flippant in answering this type of question, but humour is subjective and can land you in hot water.

If you really can't think of an answer, ask if you can return to it later in the conversation (and don't forget to do so).

Illegal questions

You likely won't encounter illegal questions during your medical-school interviews. Just in case, though, here are some examples of illegal questions in Canada:

How old are you?

Where were you born?

What's your religion?

What's your sexual orientation?

Are you married?

I see you're wearing an engagement ring. Are you getting married soon?

Do you have children or plan to have children?

What's wrong with your leg? (or any questions about physical ability)

> **INSIDER INSIGHT**
> I have not been part of a medical-school interview where an illegal question was asked. However, I have been part of employment interviews where they were asked (including when hiring physicians). So, it can happen.

I don't believe that people usually ask illegal questions with malicious intent. That doesn't excuse these questions, of course, but I think the questions can come from bumbling attempts to get information that either isn't relevant or isn't captured in the way the questions are stated.

STRATEGIES FOR ILLEGAL QUESTIONS

You might answer the question. It's your decision whether you answer an illegal question. Bear in mind that sometimes, if you answer an initial illegal question, it gives the interviewer permission to continue on in that vein and that might not be something that works in your favour (e.g., "Oh, so you're getting married this summer? So, you plan to take time off from medical school? You plan to have children soon, too? How will you accomplish that while in medical school?").

You might refuse to answer the question. This is your right. However, it can also be quite difficult to do something that feels so confrontational, during your interview (e.g., "I'm wondering what information you're looking for with this question, because I understand this question is not allowed").

You might sidestep or rephrase the question. This strategy allows you (and them) to note that the question is inappropriate, but also gives them another chance to realize their mistake and take back the question (or ask what they were really trying to get at in the first place). This might sound something like:

> "I assume you're asking about my religion because you're wondering if I can work shifts on Saturdays and Sunday. I understand this is part of the profession, so yes I can." (Note that this doesn't reveal what religion you practise, if any.)

Or:

> "I think it would be very difficult to balance children with medical school. My career is extremely important to me and I am committed to giving it my full attention." (Note that this doesn't reveal whether you do or don't have children or plan to have children.)

If you are asked an illegal question, or wondering whether a question you were asked was illegal, you may be able to appeal your interview. I would recommend talking with your career centre to get their advice. They may even be able to speak with the medical school involved, without identifying you initially, so you can figure out how or if to proceed.

Interview formats

Interview formats are constantly undergoing refinement and evolution. When I first started coaching students, most medical-school interviews were panel interviews or one-on-one interviews. There were even group interviews (where more than one applicant was interviewed at the same time). Today, medical schools use multiple mini-interviews, which is the most common format by far, and panel interviews, which a few schools continue to use.

Multiple mini-interviews

MMIs were developed at McMaster University and have since been adopted by most other medical schools across Canada.

Here's a typical set-up for MMIs. Candidates rotate through eight to twelve stations (or rooms). At each station, candidates have two minutes to read a question, prompt, or scenario. Candidates then begin the station, and have eight minutes to deal with the question, prompt, or scenario. A bell rings when the eight minutes have elapsed. Candidates then go to the next station. They get a break after rotating through half the stations.

The good news about the MMI format is that mistakes you make at any of the stations stay at those stations as you complete your mini-interviews. Say you completely fail at a station—interviewers at the next stations will not know about that: you start fresh with each station. The challenge is that you have to make new connections at every station, and keep up your energy as you go along.

Many students worry about the MMI format. From what I have seen, the questions posed during MMIs are not different from what you would encounter in any other interview format, but the aspect of timing makes the questions a little different. Many students worry about not completing an answer in eight minutes, or completing an answer before the eight minutes are up.

As with any other interview format, some questions will likely require longer answers, and some shorter answers. I can imagine that not every candidate would finish responding in the allotted time at a few stations. It may feel odd to you to get cut off mid-sentence, but it's likely a routine occurrence for the interviewers. I wouldn't worry, unless you find it happening at **every** station. In that case, you may need to edit your responses slightly.

If you are done talking before the eight minutes have elapsed, the interviewer may have follow-up questions for you, or they may not. Again, it would depend on the station. If you complete an answer before the allotted time, you will likely sit quietly while the interviewer, perhaps, catches up on notes.

It would make sense to me, given how little writing is involved in many medical-school applications these days, that MMIs might include a writing station. You may want to practise answering a question or prompt in writing within eight minutes.

MMI STRATEGIES

My experience has shown me that students are most nervous about the timing and structure of MMI-format interviews. This is something you can easily practise—by yourself, or with friends or advisors. Simply use a timer to practise reading a prompt within two minutes. Then, set the timer again for eight minutes as you answer.

When you practise with others, have them listen to your responses. Have them assess your responses for clarity of thought, logical presentation, and clear progression. Practise with other people who are applying to medical school. Take turns being the interviewer. Listening to how other people answer can be extremely helpful in boosting your own interview effectiveness.

> **ASK YOURSELF**
>
> Am I **always** done **way** before the eight minutes? Do I need to consider adding more information in my answers?
>
> Am I always being cut off by the buzzer? Do I need to edit a bit more?
>
> Am I using the two minutes of preparation effectively? How can I get a plan in place during this time?

I always advise candidates to introduce themselves in each and every MMI station. This makes sense to me, because the MMI format simulates a medical clinic, in many ways. Physicians at clinics, every time they enter an examining room, have to establish rapport, figure out who's there and why, and so on. If I were doing this type of interviewing, I would partly be assessing these aspects of a candidate (although at a level that is reasonable to expect from someone who is not yet a physician). I don't think that introducing yourself each and every time will score against you, and it just might help your cause.

> **INSIDER INSIGHT**
>
> While you are spending the two minutes reviewing the question or prompt, list the major points that you need to consider, in point form, in your head. Then, you can start the answer by outlining that "framework" and you will have a bit of a map to follow. It also helps the listener know where you are going with your answer.

Panel interviews

Panel interviews normally involve more than one interviewer. In medical-school interviewing, panels often have two interviewers: a faculty member (sometimes an MD, sometimes not) and a medical student (often second- or third-year). When I was doing medical-school interviewing, I was a third person in that group: the community member.

The good news about panel interviews is that you have some time to create a rapport with the interviewers. You have some time to calm down a bit from your initial nervous intensity. You can help interviewers develop a good sense of who you are, over several questions and a period of time (often thirty to forty minutes). The bad news is that if you stumble badly, it can feel difficult to recover.

I recall a PhD candidate we interviewed. Her answers were extremely verbose and even with prompting (e.g., "Please tell us briefly..."), she was unable to be more succinct. Had she been in an MMI format, each interviewer might not have noticed this as an overwhelming tendency, but the impression was compounded with us because we sat with her for forty-five minutes.

PANEL-INTERVIEW STRATEGIES

As with any other type of format, practising your answers out loud will help you and others see how logical and clear you sound, and whether you address the question or prompt. Try recording yourself answering a question on your voicemail. In addition to the structure and content of what you say, listen for how many "likes," "umms," and "aahs" punctuate your speech: try to reduce these a bit, if you can. Slow your speech down, if you are a fast speaker, to be sure that everyone can understand you. If you speak slowly, you may have to speed up slightly to ensure you use the allotted time effectively.

Even if everyone doesn't look friendly on the panel, try to maintain good eye contact with all the panelists, not just those who seem to "like" you. It's natural to focus slightly more on the person asking a question, so if the panelists are taking turns, you might find yourself gravitating more toward the asker. Remember to include the other panelists a bit, too.

If you are given water, be careful about nervous habits such as peeling the label off the bottle, clicking the lid repeatedly, and so on. It's likely not a deal breaker, but it can be distracting.

INSIDER INSIGHT

Show your mental work. If you simply leap to an answer, it doesn't allow interviewers to see what you have considered and learn how you approach problems or situations. Just like in elementary-school math, you may at least get partial points for your mental work!

Combined-format interviews

Some medical schools use a combination of MMI format and panel format for their interviews. Because of limited time, I expect that each of these formats is shorter than if they comprised the entire interview (e.g., four MMI stations instead of eight, plus a twenty-minute panel instead of a thirty-minute panel). In combined-format interviews, the good and bad news about both MMIs and panels apply, but I think the combined format might give applicants opportunities they would not have had if undergoing only one type of interview format.

STRATEGIES FOR COMBINED-FORMAT INTERVIEWS

Review the strategies for MMI and panel interviews earlier in this chapter. You also might want to think about which format appeals to you more—or where you can showcase your particular strengths. Sometimes shy people are very nervous about MMIs because they have to meet a new stranger in every room. The panel portion of a combined-format interview might help these people shine, on balance. Likewise, students with outgoing personalities might thrive in the MMI section and do less well in the panel section, where they may (slightly) weary a panel. There are potential opportunities for each type of person in the combined-interview format.

One-on-one interviews

I mention this format briefly because it has been used in Canada in the past. However, I have not heard of it in recent years. That doesn't mean it won't make a reappearance, though. A former medical-school hopeful I know, who interviewed at the University of British Columbia years ago, enjoyed the one-on-one format. Her interview involved only her and one faculty member—I believe it was a history professor—in a room. She felt that she could connect with one person much more naturally than with a panel (which was the predominant format at the time), and she was successful in gaining admission. She received no offers from the two other medical schools where she interviewed.

Many schools outside Canada have their recruiters or faculty conduct one-on-one interviews with candidates. This might be done in person or online. While you might like the idea of a single interviewer, the bad news about the one-on-one format is that if you are not able to connect or communicate effectively with that interviewer, your chance might be over. The same strategies for answering interview questions that apply in all other formats apply in this format: show your mental work, be clear and concise, work logically through your points, help the interviewer see your approach.

A caution about practising for interviews

Practice can help you overcome normal but incapacitating nervousness, give you strategies to deal with all kinds of different questions, and help you realize where your strengths and weaknesses lie. But, beware of overpractising.

I have encountered a few students who practised so much, and got so much well-meaning but critical feedback, that they lost all confidence. Overpractice can also sometimes create a demeanour that is almost too polished or slick, leading interviewers to wonder if they are really seeing the true candidate.

Interviewers are assessing qualities that the other elements of your application don't fully reveal. You want to show the best version of yourself during interviews, which means you still need to be **yourself**. I believe this is where interview success lies.

How to dress for interviews

Doctors don't usually work on Bay Street, so you don't need to wear a three-piece pin-stripe suit to your medical-school interview. However, you do want to dress appropriately for the occasion, and many students **do** choose to wear something resembling a suit. Decide what works best for you. Here are some basic goals to keep in mind when considering your medical-school interview outfit:

- Look tidy, professional, and competent.
- Feel confident, professional, and like the best version of yourself.
- Be somewhat memorable, but not distracting.

Many applicants wear business dress—that is, something you would see in a fairly formal office environment. Many students wear suits and ties. Others wear dresses, or dress

INSIDER INSIGHT

If you are borrowing clothes, wear them around your house to check for comfort, fit, and cleanliness. This ensures you will feel your best on interview day. The same goes for new clothes: practise wearing them, so they feel like they belong to you.

pants or skirts with shirts, blouses, or dressy sweaters. Wear whatever helps you accomplish the basic goals and reassure interviewers that they could take you to see patients without embarrassment. Feel free to wear one "statement" article, such as a distinct necklace or tie. Avoid distracting your interviewers by cluttering yourself with too much makeup or too many accessories.

Be sure to do a "circle check" to ensure that all price tags under armpits, on the bottom of shoes, and down the back of trouser legs have been removed. (I have seen more than one applicant with a price tag attached to them!) Stand up and sit down several times, so you can note any gapes or buttons that you need to wrestle with.

The interview venue will normally have a spot for you to stow items such as coats, boots, and suitcases, while you are in your interview.

Finally, avoid fragrances such as perfume, cologne, and scented body sprays. You will often be in small rooms, where they overpower, or on hospital property, where fragrances are damaging to some people.

Socials after interviews

Many medical schools offer social evenings or tours as part of their interview invitation. While you are not required to attend these events, you may find them useful as a way to learn more about the program, students, faculty, and location to which you might be headed. As far as I know, social events are not scored—however, that doesn't mean you won't be making an impression on the people you meet. My top tips are:

- Avoid drinking alcohol, if possible. If you do drink, be moderate, because nervousness tends to exacerbate the effects of alcohol.

- Prepare a few open-ended questions that will help you start conversations and convey interest. For example, "What do you like best about being in this program?" or "I've heard the skiing in this region is great. Can you tell me more?"

- Prepare an introduction that you can use when you meet people. Keep it brief and avoid being too "sales-y." A good start might be your name, where you're going to school or where you're from, and some information about your program. It's always nice to end with, "And you?" It lets the other person talk and helps keep the conversation going.

- Remember that any interactions you have with a medical school—whether it's to ask questions before you apply, or set up interview dates with administrative staff, or find a room while you're visiting—can make an impression. This might sound obvious, but many applicants are not terribly polite or patient when it comes to their email, phone, or in-person interactions with people they don't think are "important" to their medical-school admission. Those people work with the decision makers you're trying to impress—decision makers who might care about your attitude toward people in general.

14

Special-category applicants

Medical schools review some applicants under special categories, which involve processes that are different from, or additional to, their standard application processes.

In some cases, it is up to you whether to apply under a special category (e.g., categories related to identity or descent)—you will need to make a personal decision for yourself. In other cases (e.g., international students and graduate students), you will be required to apply under that category and submit additional documentation.

If you choose or are required to apply under a special category, make sure you submit all the necessary documentation for the category, so that your application isn't disqualified on a technicality.

Indigenous applicants and applicants of African descent

If you identify as Indigenous or of African descent, you can choose to apply to medical school under a special category that acknowledges your identity. Unlike other special categories, which I describe next, these special categories are not compulsory: the decision to apply under one is up to you. Medical schools often reserve spots—not many—for candidates applying under these special categories.

Many medical schools encourage applications from Indigenous students and students of African descent due to critical shortages of physicians with these identities, and to address the health-care needs of Indigenous populations and populations of African descent in Canada.

If you decide to submit as a special-category applicant because you identify as Indigenous or of African descent, you can expect to provide some or all of the following documentation:

- a letter in which you cite your ancestry and specific affiliation, request consideration under the special category, provide biographical information, and describe reasons for wanting to become a physician
- proof of ancestry
- if you are Indigenous, a letter of support from an individual representing the Indigenous community to which you belong
- if you are of African descent, a personal essay highlighting why you have chosen to apply as a special-category candidate, which will be reviewed by faculty of African descent at that university

Given the limited number of spots at some medical schools for students in these special categories, it is probably strategic to contact schools to ask how applying under these special categories might affect you. For example:

Are there any implications about being admitted under these special categories? Advantages? Disadvantages?

If I am not accepted as a special-category applicant, can I still be accepted as a noncategory applicant? (This is particularly relevant for schools that use a different process—as opposed to an additional process—to assess special-category students.)

As with every part of the application process, you may choose to seek advice from people you trust, or your career or guidance centre, on whether to apply and how to pursue additional documentation.

I have worked with students who have successfully applied under each of these categories.

Other special categories

Unlike the special categories available for students who identify as Indigenous or of African descent, some special categories are compulsory. In other words, if you fit the category, you must apply under it. Medical schools assess candidates in these special categories with processes that are additional to their standard application processes.

Graduate students

Many medical schools request that graduate students (current or past) submit additional documentation along with their application. This may include some or all of the following:

- a CV
- additional letters of reference (e.g., from a research graduate supervisor or your program director)
- a letter confirming your expected completion date, if you are currently enrolled in a graduate program

A very few medical schools grant graduate students a tiny bonus to their GPA when they apply. This is usually not enough to compensate for an undergraduate GPA that doesn't meet the standard of the applicant pool.

However, as a graduate student, your application might go in a separate evaluation "pile," because of these additional documents. If that is the case, you may receive a more holistic review as a candidate. Some students I have worked with felt this helped them gain admission to medical school.

Students pursing combined programs

Examples of combined programs include MD/PhD and MD/MSc. These programs integrate intense scientific training with medical school. Students who apply to these programs are preparing for clinician-scientist roles in academic medicine (roles that combine research, teaching, and clinical work in connection with a university).

Students need to meet the minimum criteria for each program separately. They also submit additional documents that may include some or all of the following:

- a letter of intent outlining reasons for wishing to pursue a combined program, and including information about personal and research experience
- an academic CV
- additional letters of reference from people who can comment on your research potential and ideas

There are many combinations of degrees that I have seen students undertake in conjunction with a doctor of medicine. For example, many students decide to start a master of science, or a master of education, or a master of policy studies while in medical school (or after). Some programs may require you to apply at the same time as you enter medical school, while others allow you to apply and start later. I worked with a student doing a law degree at the same time as his medical degree: his goal was to work in forensics. Some combined degrees have formal recognition, but other degree combinations are also possible. If you think this might be for you, see what you can find out about the topics that interest you.

International students

Some students attend Canadian universities as international students (i.e., they are not Canadian citizens or permanent residents). If you are an international student, you may have come from another country during your current degree or you may have completed high school in Canada. Either way, if you are applying to Canadian medical schools, you face significant challenges with admission. This is because most medical schools in Canada have no spots, or only spots numbering in the single-digits, allocated for international students. So the very strenuous admission criteria all students face are even more strenuous for international students. The University of Toronto is among the few schools that currently accepts international students. If you are applying under this category, check for updates on admissions for international students at each medical school during your year of application.

Military applicants

I haven't seen a military applicant in a few years. These are applicants who are currently employed and serving as members of the Canadian Armed Forces. These applicants come forward when the Canadian Armed Forces decides it needs more physicians—that is, if the applicant wishes to remain in the military. I know of people who have retired from or left the military to apply to medical school, which means they were no longer considered in this special category because they were no longer part of the Canadian Armed Forces. (It also meant they could apply when they wanted to.)

If you are currently serving, you will need to check with your commanding officer, and possibly your career manager, about pursuing a medical degree. Medical-school graduates in this category remain part of the military and work with military patients only.

A note about applying in French versus English

Medical schools do not have special categories related to language of learning (English or French). If you speak both languages, though, you might have options that work sort of like categories.

A few medical schools run programs in both English and French. You apply to the program in the language you wish to study—one or the other. I have worked with students who have applied to the French-language program at the University of Ottawa, for example, and the English-language program at McGill University. They applied and were interviewed in French at the University of Ottawa, and applied and were interviewed in English at McGill University.

One Ontario student I worked with felt she had a better chance of getting accepted if she applied to the French-language program at University of Ottawa: she surmised that there might be fewer French-speaking applicants for those spots. I don't know whether her surmise was correct, but she did get accepted in the French-language program and completed her MD in French.

PART III

ADDITIONAL STRATEGIES AND SPECIAL CIRCUMSTANCES

Read this section to develop a strategy that works for your unique situation.

15

Strategies for high school students

If you are reading this in high school, well done for being so proactive! There are lots of steps you can take at this stage to help prepare you for a possible application to medical school. High school is a great time to start testing the fit of many possible careers, including medicine. When you start this early, you can build useful experience in a slow and steady way, which spreads out the "work" and stress of career planning and application preparation. By the time you arrive at application decisions and documents, you will already have much of what you need to complete the task. Reducing stress, I believe, improves your chances of success.

INSIDER INSIGHT
Thinking about becoming a doctor can be very exciting, but also very stressful. If you are in high school—or even early university—this is just the beginning of your journey, and you will want to pace yourself and ensure that you are taking care of your health and wellness along the way.

Think of yourself as your first patient: be kind and reasonable to yourself. You have lots of time, you have lots of talents. Starting with specific strategies this early can be helpful for you and your application, as long as you also realize that too much stress and intensity at this stage might **not** benefit you.

This chapter offers suggestions to help you test out significant aspects of a career as a physician, and build experience that can contribute to possible medical-school applications in the future. Choose the suggestions that make sense for you.

Building health-related experience

Most students who are contemplating medical school tend to engage in or seek out activities related to health, science, and medicine. If you aren't already doing this in a formal way, you may want to add this to your activities— even in small amounts.

> **ASK YOURSELF**
> If I'm not involved with "health stuff" now, why would I be interested in it as a physician?
> How will I show that I understand some of the good, bad, and ugly about being a doctor?

In addition to general experience in health-related activities, it's also important to be able to show that you understand some specifics of the role of physician. Your volunteer job might involve bringing juice to patients, which is helpful to patients, but not the type of task that physicians generally do. However, this job can still give you a useful insider look: while you are bringing people juice, be observant, ask appropriate questions, and try to gain as many insights into why *physician* is the best role for you.

Examples of health-related activities include:

- **Volunteering in a clinical setting:** Look for opportunities in settings such as hospitals, doctors' offices, nursing homes, day cares, health units, first-aid clinics, programs for people with disabilities, and support programs for people with specific diseases and disorders (e.g., Alzheimer disease, epilepsy, diabetes).
- **School health groups and clubs:** Join activities such as cancer relays, healthy eating advocacy programs, physical or psychological wellness clubs (e.g., suicide prevention groups, body positive clubs, antidrug campaigns).
- **Job shadowing and career-information interviewing:** This can include interviewing your family doctor or other physicians about what it's like to be a doctor; asking to follow a physician around while they do their rounds; and requesting interviews or observerships with scientists who work in clinical settings (e.g., pathologists, neuroscientists, biomedical

engineers, genetics counsellors) or other clinical practitioners (e.g., physical therapists, perfusionists, medical social workers, nurse practitioners, cardiac technologists, pulmonary technicians, radiology technologists).

> **ASK YOURSELF**
>
> Can I manage to work around bodily fluids?
>
> Do I get squeamish around intense emotion or close physical contact?
>
> What age of people do I gravitate toward?
>
> What types of medical or scientific puzzles or situations intrigue me?

It can be helpful to get **any** kind of health-related experience so that you can see if you are comfortable in these types of environments.

Of course, you will not generally be able to try on the exact role of physician as a student (even if you have a physician as a relative). Your objective should be to get experience that helps you understand **your fit** with the environments, situations, stresses, and joys of this profession, so that you can show informed choice when and if you apply to medical school. Informed choice means articulating aspects of the role of physician that engage you and that are missing from other occupations you have explored (especially clinical, scientific, or health-related occupations). If you focus **only** on the role of physician, you might not be able to make your case for why it is the **best** health-care role for you.

Building research experience

Most high school students have few opportunities to engage in research: I doubt medical schools expect much experience with research in

> **INSIDER INSIGHT**
>
> Getting some exposure to research at this stage can help you see what elements of research you really like.

high school. However, part of being a doctor is having an interest in research that might affect patients.

Many university students I speak with simultaneously apply to research positions (e.g., graduate programs or jobs) and to medical school, because they know that they like the research part of being a physician. If they don't get into medical school right away, or ever, they know research might provide a great alternate career path for them.

Or not—sometimes, exposure to research helps students understand that research is really **not** their primary interest. This can help cement a decision to pursue a more clinical role, such as doctor or something else.

As you can see, research experience can benefit you, whether you end up applying to medical school or not.

If you do apply to medical school, you are often required to list any formal research experience you have (as opposed to small projects you may have done as part of course work). This requirement may reflect that research is part of medical training, so medical schools may want to assess your motivation to engage in research. Or, the requirement may reflect that physicians need to stay up to date with research that affects their specialties and patients, so medical schools may want to assess whether you already have this inclination, which would be helpful in your future career as a doctor.

As a high school student, it can be challenging to get formal research experience. Here are some ideas:

- **Summer jobs in research:** Some research units at hospitals and universities hire summer students to assist with basic research tasks. Others enlist volunteers. These roles can be difficult to get as a high school student, but may be worth asking about, especially if you know anyone who works in a lab or research situation. Even if you're washing test tubes, you'll get valuable insights into the workings of this type of environment.

- **Observerships in research:** This involves "shadowing" a researcher for a period to see what their work entails. To arrange an observership, you need to contact labs or research units doing work that interests you. You might start by speaking with the people who work under senior researchers in these labs or units. These people include PhD candidates or postdoctoral fellows, and they are often more accessible than senior researchers. Check medical-school websites for information about departments, people, body parts, and diseases that interest you. Most researchers have web pages that describe their projects, papers, and interests.

- **Volunteering as a research subject:** Joining a research study as a subject can be enlightening and is often very accessible to high school students. Many researchers seek participants that fit particular criteria. I know students who have taken part in allergy studies (one student made some money by spending his weekends in an allergy lab, where he was exposed to ragweed and treated for his reactions), cardiac studies, sexual health studies, music studies, bicycling studies, sleep studies, and psychology studies, just to name a few. If you are younger than eighteen, you will likely require a parent's permission to participate.

- **Independent research study:** You can request an independent study from a high school or university instructor. If you have a particular topic of interest, ask if it's possible for you to do "directed readings," possibly concluding with a report. Most medical schools don't consider projects within the regular requirements of a course as "research," but an independent study over and above regular requirements can provide a formal and autonomous way to demonstrate research experience and interest.

Pursuing community service

In high school especially, it's normal for your community-service activities to take place in and around your school. If you are thinking about medical school in the future, you might want to add one or two activities that engage a larger community. A larger community could include:

- a cultural community (e.g., Filipino, African, Francophone)
- an identity community (e.g., bisexual people, new immigrants, a visible minority, inmates)
- an age community (e.g., teenagers, mature students, the elderly)
- a geographic community (e.g., rural Nova Scotians, inner-city residents)
- a socioeconomic community (e.g., teens with single parents, low-income families)
- a health community (e.g., teens with Crohn disease, cancer survivors)
- an interest community (e.g., a basketball league, a string ensemble, a science-fiction fan club)

Try to seek out one opportunity that allows you to demonstrate a need you've seen in your community where you initiate solutions. For example, one student I worked with noticed that her cultural community had a high rate of suicide, yet there were no mental health supports specific to that community's youth. She started a program in her region, which she has since extended to high schools across the country. Another student noticed that many high school girls faced financial obstacles when buying a dress for prom or graduation. She started a charitable organization to accept donated dresses. It offered students who wanted a dress a nonjudgemental day of pampering to get their hair done, try dresses on, and choose a dress for free.

These types of activities can demonstrate a host of valuable attributes including initiative, perseverance, business acumen, compassion, commitment, time management, advocacy, social justice, and more. They are impressive because you didn't simply join—you initiated and created.

Choose activities that suit your interests and that you feel strongly about. Strong feelings often reveal passions that might turn into a community activity.

ASK YOURSELF

What do I argue with people about?

What do I wish my community had that it doesn't currently have?

What makes me sad?

What do people know me for?

What do I know a lot about, or wish I could know a lot about?

What issues have touched me?

Building other experience

Preparing for the possibility of medical school is about more than gathering activities like eggs in a basket. It also involves reflecting on formal and informal ways you live your life. Many students gain incredible experiences working on their family farm, or in their family corner store or restaurant. Others assist in taking care of live-in grandparents or siblings with disabilities. I've met students who spend a lot of their free time earning money simply to keep themselves and their families afloat. They can't afford to buy textbooks, so they use the library. Many students have immigrated to Canada without their parents, and have lived on their own (or in a stranger's family) while attending Canadian high school or university. Some students report that their parents' hardships or journeys have deeply affected them, and they have grown up with a profound sense of wanting to "give back." I've also met students who live with illness or disease, or endure speech or language struggles, mental health disorders, or learning or physical disabilities. One student I worked with spoke about a basketball injury that resulted in knee surgery, significant time off from the game, and a reexamination of who she was "without basketball."

You don't need a dramatic tragedy to convey these kinds of experiences successfully. Think about your own story, and if and how it has affected your desire to become a physician.

ASK YOURSELF

Who am I because of my experiences? What has motivated me along the way?

What have been my biggest challenges or failures? What have I struggled with?

When have I triumphed?

Building maturity

Maturity is hard to quantify. In my opinion, medical schools see maturity in someone who:

- understands themselves fairly well (at a level appropriate to their age): their motivations, their strengths and weaknesses
- understands the career of physician fairly well: the excitement, the challenges
- balances confidence and humility: understands that their successes are not wholly theirs, but the culmination of privilege, circumstances, luck, and skill

Maturity is difficult to teach or coach. Yet, students often ask me how they can convey this in their applications and interviews. In thinking about this, I believe that self-reflection can be a large part of conveying maturity. You don't simply talk about what you did—you talk about what you learned from it and how it is carrying you forward.

Here are a few of my ideas about how to get there:

- **Listen to others:** Whom do you admire? How do they describe themselves and their accomplishments? Do they boast? Do they quietly contribute?

- **Listen to yourself:** When do you take sole credit versus sharing credit? Do you use the pronoun *I* more than *we*? Do you think of yourself as "motivated, hardworking, and powerful" or as "fortunate"?
- **Seek feedback:** What do others say about you? Ask people who love you (parents, family, friends), and people who don't necessarily love you, but who know you (e.g., employers, volunteer supervisors, teachers and professors, coaches). What do they see as your strengths and weaknesses? How does this resonate with what you know about yourself? How can you build on current strengths and mitigate weaknesses? What advice do others suggest for building maturity?
- **Interact with people who are not like you:** Princess Diana encouraged her sons to engage with people "not like them"—people with HIV, people without privilege, people who faced great stigma. I believe engaging others this way fosters understanding, compassion, gratitude, and a whole host of attributes that, to me, lead to maturity. If you are only engaged with people from your geographic location, culture, age group, socioeconomic group, and identity, I believe you limit your opportunities for growth. And growth often results in maturity.

Building communication skills

Many students applying to medical school are engaged in scientific programs and sometimes favour activities that don't involve much writing or speaking. If that seems true for you, don't lose sight of this fact: the application process for medical school is based on written and verbal communication. Here are some ideas to build your communication skills:

- **Practise writing regularly:** Look for opportunities through academic work and creative pursuits. Consider taking a writing-based course to keep your skills up. Craft editorials for news outlets on issues that have meaning for you. Start a blog or write a blog post about topics that interest you.
- **Speak with others:** Do this even if you are shy. Practise explaining complicated concepts in simple ways. Practise talking with people who are not "like you"—for example,

adults and elderly people, professionals you admire, bloggers you follow, small children, people whose first language is not the same as yours.

- **Record yourself:** If you are nervous about speaking, try talking to yourself on voicemail or video. Watch for eye contact and filler words such as "like" and "ummmm."
- **Engage in public speaking:** Speaking in public is a very common fear. Try answering more questions in class, doing presentations, doing videos of yourself, or teaching something to others. Some students join Toastmasters, which has local branches across the country to help people learn and practise public-speaking skills.

Next steps

High school is long. By the time you reach university, and possibly graduate school, and possibly a medical-school application, your experiences from high school can be hard to remember. I suggest finding a place (electronic or paper) where you can record notes about your activities as you do them or just after you complete them. Some ideas about what to record include:

- the dates, organization, and your role for each activity
- the name and contact information of someone who can verify that you actually did the activity (not a family member)
- reflections on the best parts and the most-challenging parts of the activity, and any accomplishments you realized
- names and contact information of people who might provide you a reference (keep in touch with them at least once a year to update them on your progress and activities)

This should not take much time, and is extremely helpful when it comes to later tasks such as writing résumés for jobs, completing applications for university (including, sometimes, application essays), and applying to medical school and other programs.

Communicating your experiences

It can be challenging to effectively communicate what you did and what you learned. You want to be honest and positive about your activities, but that's not always easy. Try some of these strategies:

- Review job descriptions, volunteer orientation sheets, course outlines, or any other information associated with your activities. Reflect on the best and most-challenging aspects of your role in each activity. What, if any, accomplishments did you realize? Make point-form notes.

- Focus your writing on actions. Using active verbs to start point-form sentences can be helpful. For example, "mentored fourteen rugby players weekly as team captain" has more action, specificity, and clarity than "rugby team captain for two seasons." Check out chapter 9 of this resource for more tips on writing.

- Ask others you trust to read your notes. Do they get a clear picture of what you contributed, learned, and accomplished? Parents, physicians, mentors, guidance counsellors, and career counsellors can all provide helpful assistance in this process.

16

You didn't get in: Now what?

It is understandable that this is a chapter you might want to avoid. Most people prefer to think about positive results and not contemplate the scary or negative "what ifs."

Everyone should read this chapter, though. At the very least, you should read it because it might help you answer the common interview question, "What will you do if you don't get in this time?"

You should also read this chapter because most applicants **don't** get in on their first application to medical school. And when you don't get in, you need to decide whether to forge ahead with applying again or forge ahead on another path. No matter what you decide, I encourage you to avoid getting "stuck." I have worked with students who persist in applying year after painful year, not progressing in any other career directions while they hope to get into medical school. In one extreme example, I worked with a student who was on his tenth application. His autobiographical sketch revealed that his career plans hadn't moved forward in those ten years, and I believe this became a major obstacle to his admission. On the other hand, I know students who have persisted, consistently improving their applications and interviews with each application cycle, and have ultimately succeeded in entering medical school in Canada.

Keep moving forward. Being a physician might be your dream job, but it's not the only job that can offer you success and happiness. Showing that *physician* is the **best** fit for you, rather than the only fit for you, is a good step for your mental health, career, and subsequent applications.

Not getting accepted is normal

If you are reading this chapter because you didn't get accepted to medical school, you need to know that this is a very normal situation.

> **INSIDER INSIGHT**
>
> **Most** applicants do not succeed in gaining admission to medical school in Canada on their first try.

Some statistics indicate that less than fourteen percent of first-time applicants are successful in Canada. There are simply too many qualified applicants and too few spots. Rejection does not mean that you are a "bad" candidate or not meant for this career. The overwhelming majority of students I work with are good medical-school candidates—they're not deluding themselves. Rejection usually means that you should revisit your application strategy (e.g., how many schools to apply to, which locations, and so on), or your application elements (e.g., your GPA, your supplemental materials), to see where you could improve. Often, however, your application strategy and elements are sound: you didn't get in because you were applying in a year with a very strong applicant pool. This meant you were slightly below the cutoff for the number of offers the schools could make.

When I interviewed students as part of a medical-school admissions panel, I found this heart-breaking every year. Candidates offered interviews are, in my experience, excel-lent, but medical schools inter-

> **INSIDER INSIGHT**
>
> Medical schools often have more excellent candidates than available spots. This means they can only give offers to the "most excellent" of the excellent.

view far more candidates than they can accept.

This may be the first time you have failed to achieve a goal that you set for yourself. For many medical-school applicants, that is the case. As a group, you tend to be very high achievers who, by and large, attain your goals. It can therefore come as a big shock when you don't get an offer from a medical school after doing everything "right." In my experience, a difficult part of this process is that you can do everything "right" and still not get accepted.

Not getting accepted hurts

I encourage you to acknowledge the disappointment, which can often be extreme, when rejection occurs.

"Failing" at something like this, especially if it is your first time, can take a toll on your self-esteem, your sense of identity ("But, I've always been very smart!"), and your confidence. It can feel embarrassing to admit that you didn't get in, especially to people who have helped you or known your goal. It might feel as if everyone expected you to succeed, as you have always done in the past. Others might not have any idea of the competition to get in, or the many steps involved in the process. Rejection might cause you to experience self-doubt with thoughts like "maybe I'm not good enough" or "I did something wrong."

Spend some time recovering from the blow. It's okay to "wallow" for a while and feel sorry for yourself. Let others take care of you and offer sympathy. Consider seeking help from professionals.

> **INSIDER INSIGHT**
> A kind of grieving process can take hold in this situation. You might feel jealous or angry about people who get accepted. I've often heard students remark, "They got in and I always had better grades than them."

It can be very puzzling to understand why you didn't get accepted: the reasons are not always very clear, even on analysis. This can be frustrating for the problem-solving part of you, who wants to fix whatever went wrong and carry on. Your supporters might offer well-intentioned advice about how to improve your chances next time. You might not be ready to hear that yet—so you might need to let them know that, right now, you just need some space to digest the bad news.

It will be some time before you can reapply (if you decide to), so allow yourself time to process this disappointment and start to recover from it.

Why were you not accepted?

Depending on your personality, you might want to "figure out what went wrong" immediately after your rejection. I encourage you to wait a bit. If you do this too soon, you won't be as objective as you can be later on. In reassessing your applications, you also might want to seek perspectives from others, including family, physicians, professors, mentors, and career or guidance counsellors. These people can be very helpful, both in reassuring you about where you excel and providing some insights into where you might improve.

If you decide to reapply, consider how far you got in the application process the last time. Here are common scenarios I've worked through with students:

- **Applied to many schools, got no interviews:** This may indicate that something in the student's application (e.g., GPA, MCAT score, CASPer score, or supplemental materials) did not meet the standard of the applicant pool that year.

- **Applied to a couple of schools, got no interviews:** This may indicate that the student should apply more broadly next time. It may also indicate that their application did not meet the applicant-pool standard that year, but this conclusion is harder to support, given how few programs the student applied to.

- **Got one interview, got no offer:** This might not indicate any problems with interview performance, but rather, simply, not enough available spots to offer acceptance to the student. However, it might still indicate that something about their interview performance could be revisited.

- **Got several interviews, got no offers**: This might indicate that something about the student's interview performance could be improved. However, this outcome might result from medical schools having too many "most excellent" candidates to choose from.

Many factors can play into each of these scenarios, so they are useful only to a point. Their best use might be as a starting point for you to try to strategize about what, if anything, you can improve in your next applications to medial school.

Where your application "stopped"

Some schools provide you with written feedback (with your rejection) about which part of the application process you "stopped" at. This can be very helpful, but not every school chooses to give applicants this type of information.

BEFORE INTERVIEWS

If you didn't get interviews, it can be a function of the applicant pool that year (very strong), meaning some elements of your application didn't quite clear the bar. For example, if a school interviews 500 candidates and figures out who this is by ranking the top 500 GPAs, if your GPA is not among the top 500 for that applicant pool (even though you meet the minimum required and have an excellent GPA), you might not be invited for an interview. Some medical schools judge your entire application (which includes, depending on the school, your GPA, MCAT score, CASPer score, supplemental materials, and references) against the standard set by that year's applicant pool. Other medical schools judge only certain application elements this way (e.g., only GPA or only CASPer score), which means those elements were specific obstacles in the context of that year's applicant pool.

AFTER INTERVIEWS

Every school approaches the application and interview process slightly differently, but I believe it's a very good sign if you got to the interview stage of the process. Most schools cannot realistically interview everybody who applies (25,000 people in some cases), which means that your application merited getting into at least some form of "short list" for interviews.

AFTER WAIT-LISTING

If you are wait-listed at a medical school, it means you will be offered a spot if another candidate turns it down. It is very disappointing to be wait-listed and then not get in—but, it is a very hopeful sign, too. It means you met the criteria for "mostly excellent" among the "most excellent" group, and any small improvements you can make, if you decide to apply again, could help you reach your goal.

Will you reapply?

If this is your first rejection and you still want to become a doctor, I encourage you to apply again. That is because it is so common for great applicants to face rejection the first time. Perhaps I am biased because of the work I do, but I believe that the chances for success can improve with the knowledge that comes from going through the process once (or more than once). In many cases, students learn strategies that improve their application elements and interviews the next time around.

If you decide to reapply, the next question is when.

Many students reapply the year after their first application. Some students wait a year or two, or until they finish another degree. A student I worked with was rejected at

> **ASK YOURSELF**
>
> How will I answer the question, "Why did you not get in last time and why should we accept you this time?"

the end of his undergraduate degree. He then completed a PhD, reapplied, and was accepted. In 2018, he applied to residency programs and was extremely competitive because of his maturity and the research experience he gained as a PhD student, before his MD. He also plans to become a clinician-scientist, pairing research with clinical work, so the delay due to the PhD has helped him clarify a career path.

If and when you decide to reapply, I encourage you to think about how you can show improvement and growth in your application next time.

Improving your undergraduate GPA

In some cases, it is extremely helpful to complete an undergraduate degree before applying to medical school, so that all your undergraduate grades can go toward your cumula-

> **INSIDER INSIGHT**
>
> Simply applying the year after you complete your undergraduate degree can result in an improvement in your candidacy.

tive GPA. If you applied during third or fourth year, you will have missed some of these grades. If your GPA is "on the cusp," this might have compromised your competitiveness. In the case of programs that allow you to remove a couple of lower grades or earlier credits (as the University of Toronto has allowed in the past), applying in the year after you complete your undergraduate degree can offer the same GPA boost.

You might also consider applying to programs that have an alternate GPA calculation. For example, understanding that many students have a transition to university that results in some lower grades, especially in first year, Queen's University has allowed candidates' GPAs to be calculated based on the last two years of their program, if they don't meet the applicant-pool standard in the cumulative GPA calculation. Would your last two years raise your

GPA? Don't forget: this may also have a positive effect on your competitors' grades, applying under this same calculation.

If your undergraduate GPA is complete but still not as competitive as you'd like, consider this strategy: some students take more undergraduate courses in hopes of raising their cumulative GPA. You may find many rumours about the "best" way to raise a GPA. I caution you to be sure that you get your information from the source that matters: the medical schools to which you will be applying. Factors change from year to year, and you need the most current information.

ASK YOURSELF

If you are thinking about raising your GPA by taking more undergraduate courses, think about these questions:

How many medical schools, if any, consider more undergraduate courses—after I've finished my first degree—as part of their cumulative GPA calculation? (Ask the medical schools.)

From a medical-school application perspective, is it better to take more undergraduate courses or move on to additional education (e.g., master's degree, professional degree)? (Ask the medical schools.)

How does taking additional or random undergraduate courses make my application look? Is there any negative impact? (Ask the medical schools.)

Are there undergraduate or graduate courses I could take that would help my cumulative GPA, and also give me additional career options, if I don't get into medical school? (Ask a medical school, then ask a trusted career advisor.)

Going on to further education

Many students naturally think about undertaking further education such as master's degrees, professional degrees, or postdegree programs to improve their GPA for medical school. Why would they take more undergraduate credits when they already have a completed degree?

Be careful: medical schools currently emphasize undergraduate grades very strongly. Most give you extremely little, if any, GPA benefit because of your status as a graduate student.

In addition, some medical schools consider graduate students separately from undergraduate students. Find out if this is the case at the medical schools to which you plan to apply, in the year you plan to apply, and whether they have advice on how graduate studies might work for or against you as a candidate.

Of course, graduate or professional programs offer other great benefits to you, from additional career options to additional experience. However, most graduate programs don't want to be a stepping-stone or a time killer for people really aiming for medical school. You will need to demonstrate strong commitment and focused interest to these programs.

INSIDER INSIGHT

From a career perspective, it would make sense to consider further education if it fits with your goals or interests, and if you've already completed an undergraduate degree. However, you may wish to investigate whether anything other than more *undergraduate* credits will actually benefit your application, if you feel GPA was the barrier to your medical-school admission.

Consider carefully what medical schools consider "further education," because some postdegree options such as postdegree college programs, work, volunteering, and travel, while excellent career-building options, do not count toward the GPA portion of a medical-school application. Instead, they help with the elements of applications that describe experiences and activities (e.g., autobiographical sketch, CV, résumé, references).

Improving MCAT scores

Many students write the MCAT twice. Some write it more than that. If you have received information that your MCAT score is your stumbling block and are considering rewriting, think about the following:

- **Medical schools treat repeat MCAT scores differently.** Some might average your scores, some might review the latest scores, some might review your best score. Often, medical schools see how many times you have written. How will you defend your number of attempts, if asked?

- **By trying to improve your score, you may be risking an already-decent score.** Do you have any evidence that your MCAT score was a significant obstacle in the application process?

- **It costs money and time to rewrite.** Can you afford to write it again? Can you afford not to?

- It might make sense to rewrite if a particular section of the MCAT is a problem. If you didn't meet the minimum score on that section, you didn't clear the MCAT hurdle at all.
- You might have gained useful experience from your first attempt at the test. Perhaps you can see where you could improve on your preparation or execution. You might have insights about when best to write it, so you make the most of your chance for improvement. Perhaps you could write it before your application deadlines to allow you to strategize about where to apply.

Many students I work with report that they didn't significantly improve their MCAT scores on a repeat attempt. However, some students do improve their scores, and some are able to increase scores in specific disqualifying sections (sections that some medical schools require students to pass for MCAT scores to qualify at all).

Be sure to also check that your standing MCAT score will still be eligible for the year in which you apply. The score expires (usually after three years).

Improving CASPer scores

CASPer is not currently required as part of the application process at every school, but I wonder if it will increase in popularity (in the context of interviews, this has happened with the MMI format). My sense is that, if students are able to improve their CASPer scores, improvement comes from experience with the test. On a repeat test, you already have a sense of how it works, the types of scenarios it poses, and the speed at which you need to think (and type). Additional ideas for improving include:

- Continue to practise typing, so that your speed increases. (Ability to think and type quickly can be important.)
- Practise timed writings: answer ethics questions, for example, that come out of the daily news (and time yourself).
- Review the information in chapter 11 for additional CASPer preparation strategies.

Improving your autobiographical sketch, curriculum vitae, or résumé

If you have received feedback about your supplemental materials, consider spending the time between now and your next application increasing the diversity of your experience, or gaining more experience in certain areas.

ASK YOURSELF

Does my autobiographical sketch, CV, or résumé show gaps in qualities or experiences desired by medical schools? (For example, am I lacking research experience?) What can I do to fill those gaps between now and my next application?

Did I choose the best referees? Do they still support me and my application? Do I need to review my goals and accomplishments with them before my next application, to help them write the best reference possible?

Is my autobiographical sketch, CV, or résumé written as well as it could be? Is it clear? Does it optimize the space allowed to showcase my best attributes and skills? Should I seek others' input into how it reads?

Am I showing a balance between school and other activities? Do I engage in my local and broader community? Do I show initiative in identifying and solving problems?

Is there a way to explain any "blips" or elements that might read as confusing?

When consulting others about these elements of your application, ask them to tell you what they understand about your activities and attributes. Do they understand what you want them to understand? Are they missing something important that helps you connect to being a good future medical student and doctor?

Improving interview performance

As I have mentioned, you may have gotten interviews and still not received an offer, and this is not necessarily a function of "bad" interview technique. Interviews tend to be nervous situations for everyone (including sometimes the interviewers). Some candidates find it helpful to do "mock interviews" as practice.

ASK YOURSELF

Does nervousness compromise my presentation at interviews? (Remember, it's normal to be nervous—in and of itself, nervousness is not a negative.) If I feel nervousness poses a significant obstacle to my success in interviews, what strategies have helped me calm nervousness in other situations? Can I use these strategies in a future medical-school interview?

What kind of practice would be helpful to me? For example, did I struggle with strategies for breaking down questions, speaking logically, or speaking too much or too little?

Did I show informed choice for this career? What can I do before my next interview to help show that I understand what I'm getting into?

Do I need more strategies to help deal with ethics, behavioural, or situational questions? Where can I find resources to help me?

Am I staying current with health issues local to where I'm interviewing, and in Canada and the world? Am I paying attention to current events, and can I speak to some nonheadline issues, if asked?

You can request mock or practice interviews at your guidance or career centre. These can be a helpful way to get in the "zone" of interviewing (some candidates even dress as if they were going to a real interview) and get feedback on the areas you may wish to improve. It's also a great way to practise getting nervous and overcoming those nerves.

Next steps

When you are rejected (again, I want to remind you how normal this is), you need to decide if and when you might apply again. This is a very personal decision and there is no wrong answer. A friend of mine applied three times and then, in her words, "took the hint." She was in an undergrad optometry program and became an optometrist. On reflection, she is very happy with her decision, and often comments that she prefers her lifestyle to that of her physician friends.

Another rejected student (you met him in an earlier chapter) applied to a fast-track nursing degree after first hearing about it from me. He readily admitted later that he took nursing as a way to increase his undergraduate GPA, so he could reapply to MD programs. However, once in nursing, he realized that he had been ignorant of what nurses did, really loved that role, and has remained there very happily.

Many students apply twice and get in the second time they apply.

Some students opt to go in a different direction, preferring research or some other clinical profession (e.g., nursing, physical therapy, occupational therapy, dentistry, pharmacy, X-ray technology). None of these prohibit another application to medical school in the future, and they allow students to move forward in careers that are also suitable for them—sometimes for a while, and sometimes as a permanent career choice.

ASK YOURSELF

How many times will I reapply, if any?

Is becoming a physician still my goal? Are there other careers that also make sense? For example, if I like the "working with patients" part of medicine, what other careers engage that skill? What if I like the "problem-solving" or "puzzle" part? What about if I like the "leading a team" part? (Read chapter 3 for more ideas.)

When does it make sense to reapply, if I do?

If I plan to reapply, what can I do in the meantime to move forward? How can I show medical schools improvement next time? How can I avoid stagnating in a cycle of waiting?

How could I improve my application for next time?

Could I change my strategy to improve my chances next time?

Are there other places to apply (e.g., outside my home province, outside Canada) that make sense for me?

17

How parents and other supporters can help

In my experience working with students over the past twenty years, I have noticed that applying to medical school—perhaps more than applying to any other kind of program—seems to be a family affair.

If you are a parent or person supporting someone applying to medical school now or in the future, you may already know about some of the fallout: feeling stressed on your student's behalf, losing sleep, trying to uncover "secret" strategies, wishing you could make things easier, wondering how best to be helpful.

Your support is key

Rest assured, you can be of great help to your student, simply by being there. It probably doesn't surprise you that many surveys identify parents as the number-one source of career advice for today's students. Students value your experience, your wisdom, your perspective. Perhaps they also know that you are their biggest fans and supporters of their dreams.

Students have told me that the most helpful support parents can give has these characteristics:

- It is nonjudgemental (e.g., "My parents support my career goals, whatever they may be").

- It offers help without undue pressure (e.g., "My parents want to help, but they let me decide when").
- It is realistic (e.g., "My parents reassure me about what I'm good at, and also help me strategize about my weaknesses").

Of course, as a parent or supporter, you will have your own strategies that work for you and your student. This chapter offers insights into the "most-helpful help" based on two decades of hearing students complain about and extol the people who love them. The suggestions here—though only suggestions—come from many conversations with students.

Understand the challenge

Students often report to me that they feel caught between their parents and the news. Parents who haven't been to medical school (and even those who have) hear reports that "Canada needs more doctors," which causes the parents to wonder whether it's *that* hard to get into medical school. "They don't understand how competitive it is," students say to me. Students whose parents are physicians often worry, "They don't understand how competitive it is **now**."

Other students worry about disappointing their supporters: "I've always done so well and they don't really understand that this is different." Many students feel the weight of family expectations: "I'm the first to go to university," or "I'm in Canada because I'm expected to go to medical school here," or "They have spent a lot of money getting me here—I don't want to let them down."

It is **very normal** for your always-previously-successful student to not get in the first time they apply to medical school in Canada. And it is **very normal** for students to suffer from self-doubt before, during, or after the application process: "Did I do enough? Am I good enough? Will I ever get in? What went wrong?"

Mental health agencies, in recent years, have reported stress among students in high school and university at all-time highs. I don't like that the quest for medical school feeds into this, but the reality is that applying to medical school can affect your student's well-being. I have talked with many students who haven't slept enough, are working too hard, are doing too many things, and who don't give themselves a well-deserved break when they should.

You can help them recognize that this is a long, competitive process—something to pace themselves for. Concepts you may wish to reinforce include:

- You are enough, whether you get in or not.
- Most students don't get in the first time, and I will support you however many times you apply.
- If this is your goal, I will help you in whatever way I can to achieve it.
- Taking a break to recharge will actually help you achieve this goal.
- This is a very challenging goal, and it can be tiring and frustrating. You can talk to me about it, whenever you need to.
- There is help available when you need it—at your school and here at home.

If you are new to the process of applying to medical school, or new to it as a recent task, I encourage you to read chapter 2 in this resource about what makes getting into medical school difficult.

Let your student find their own way

Applying to professional schools, such as medical schools, can come with a host of complicated implications. Being a doctor is sometimes seen, in North America and many other parts of the world, as a pinnacle career ambition. Your status as a parent or supporter of a student applying to, or attending, medical school might seem to rise as a result. Your status, if they "fail," can seem to fall as a result. It can be challenging to separate your student's goals from your own goals, ambitions, dreams, and hopes.

Sometimes, students report to me, "The only career my parents will support is doctor." Sometimes, they just say, "They really want me to be a doctor." I don't know whether this is, in fact, what their parents think. But it doesn't really matter, because it is what the students believe the parents think.

My worry, as a helping professional, is what impact this belief has on a student's stress and well-being. I also worry, as someone who has screened applicants to medical school, about the impact this belief has on a student's candidacy. How can a student demonstrate interest in and commitment to becoming a doctor if the goal is not their own, but their parent's?

I always tell students that, however they hear messages from their parents, my sense is that parents want their students to be safe and happy most of all. Regardless of how that comes across in what parents say, or how students interpret what parents say, that is *really* what parents are saying.

The next sections offer suggestions to help your student find a safe and happy route through the medical-school application process, and beyond.

Encourage academic interests

ASK YOURSELF

What are my secret and not-so-secret hopes and dreams for my student?

How does my student seem to be doing?

Does my student articulate why this goal is important to them?

Is my student seeking out information voluntarily and preparing enthusiastically toward this goal? Or does it seem like I have to push them forward?

Are there supports at school or in the community that could help my student make decisions, apply, and deal with the process?

Medical schools do not require any specific degree programs as preparation. A few medical schools specify prerequisite courses, but these courses can fit into any degree program. For example, a fine arts student can apply to many medical schools, and can apply to even more if they include in their program a few basic science courses (e.g., biology, organic chemistry). Check medical schools each year to see what, if any, prerequisites they list.

This means that you can encourage your student to take courses and programs that they are really interested in. Naturally, students thinking about medical school are often drawn to science or health-based programs such as life or health sciences, biology, psychology, chemistry, or nursing. However, many students who study engineering, geography, humanities, languages, or English also apply to medical school.

Students who are interested in their subject matter tend to do better academically. They seem to get higher grades, and this can be very helpful in the medical-school admissions process.

In this way, it's practical to advise your student to "study what you love," bearing in mind any specific prerequisite courses for particular medical schools.

Remember: they will likely apply more than once (and this is normal)

Some statistics indicate that less than fourteen percent of first-time applicants to Canadian medical schools are accepted. That means that it's very, very normal for your highly talented, extremely smart, caring, contributing student to **not get in** on their first try.

I can't emphasize this enough, because, as a group, you are not people who are used to paying attention to the depressing statistics. Your student has always succeeded at

INSIDER INSIGHT

The pressure to overcome the rejection-rate statistic for first-time applicants to medical school can be immense. I recommend relieving some of that pressure by reassuring your student that **getting rejected the first time is the rule and not the exception.** If you stick to this message all the way through the process, you can help your student see rejection as a natural part of applying to medical school, instead of a huge failure when it happens.

every challenge. They may succeed with this challenge—but if they don't, it doesn't mean that they, or you, have failed.

It can be very hard to wrap your head around the fact that failure on the first try is likely, but I think it's important that you do. Your student may seek your support and reassurance when they find the application process difficult, and if they are rejected in the end. It can be hard to convince them that it's normal to be rejected, if the first time they hear that message is **after** they've been rejected.

Encourage thinking about additional career paths

From a mental health perspective as well as for the application process, I recommend students consider additional career paths. When completing an application or interview for medical school, knowledge of additional career paths can show that a student is making an informed choice about the role of physician, and not simply a choice expected of them or based on vague notions that lack insight into the day-to-day tasks of physicians.

Exploring additional careers also helps students clarify alternate, appealing paths to take, if they don't gain admission to medical school. Students can pursue these alternate paths as they reapply to medical school (if they choose to reapply). Alternate paths allow students to progress in another career, in case they change their mind about medical school or don't ever gain admission. It helps students view other careers as "also great," rather than "less than great," if medical school doesn't work out.

Read chapter 3 for ideas on exploring other career options.

Offer support if spirits (or grades) flag

Students thinking about medical school can be (justifiably) intense and hard on themselves. My experience with university students, and even some high school students, is that "academic blips" are hardest for more-informed students. Not getting into the university of their choice, facing (common) dips in first-year university grades, and digesting their (often less-than-stellar) first exam results can cause significant distress to students. University may present the first time that students take classes with others who value education highly, do well in school, and strive for excellence in ways similar to them. This can dent their self-confidence: their once-special attributes now seem almost ordinary, everywhere they look. As a parent, you may or may not be aware that this is happening to your student, especially if they are away from home.

Students in university are treated as adults, and you will likely not be notified about their grades, problems, or trips to the doctor. This can leave some parents feeling very "out of the loop" and worried. I'm not a parent myself, so I asked some parents I have worked with for strategies they used with their students who were thinking about medical school. Their suggestions (which I encourage you to incorporate or ignore, as they fit your own parenting style) included:

- Remind students that they might need to "fight" for grades, if they feel they were marked unfairly.
- Suggest that students keep an ongoing list of their activities and contacts, starting in high school. One parent suggested that parents take ownership of this for their students, since the students are so busy. I think that's a personal decision for every family to make. My career-counsellor bias is that it's important for students to take on this chore themselves, so that they have some chance to reflect on their activities (which is helpful for later job and other applications).
- Reinforce aspects of your student that are **not** about academics. Consider reminding them about the person they are as a

whole, and not just as a student, and how much you value and believe in that person.

- Consider taking them out of their academic environment for a break once in a while. Going to lunch, or driving down for a weekend so they can show you their new town, can help your student decompress from the school environment.
- Beware of false friends, rumours, and fearmongering.
- Help your student think strategically about everything they do, from high school forward. Help them consider, as they choose options and seek experience, "How does this help me in my bid for medical school?"
- Consider keeping your student's career goals somewhat quiet. For your student, not getting in can feel more like failure when everyone knows that was their goal.
- Remind your student about school or on-campus supports available to them: academic advisors, study help, career advisors, mental health programs, and so on. These supports are usually free of charge, and have very qualified staff experienced in working with the student population.

Refer to school and campus resources and supports

Many school and campus resources are available to your student. Parents of high school students may be able to connect with them directly. Parents of university students will need to encourage the students themselves to reach out. This section offers suggestions on where to start.

For academic questions and issues, start with:

- teachers, professors, teaching assistants
- academic advisors, undergraduate assistants, undergraduate chairs (in the faculty or department associated with your student's program)
- graduate assistants and graduate chairs (if your student is in a master's or PhD program)
- learning strategies departments (for help with study skills and more)
- writing centres (for help with development of writing skills)
- accessibility services (for academic accommodations)

For career exploration, and help with application and interview strategies, start with:

- guidance departments (high school)
- family physicians
- career centre staff (university)
- professors, teachers, teaching assistants
- faculty or department assistants (in the faculty or department associated with your student's program)

For wellness, health, and mental health, start with:

- school nurse, doctor, social worker, counsellor
- student wellness services
- residence floor advisor or don
- school health promotion programs (e.g., drinking cessation, antianxiety programs, healthy eating programs)
- any advisor: academic, career, guidance, faculty
- recreation and fitness programs, athletic teams
- campus chaplain

This is by no means a complete list, but I hope it will help you ask for and find the people who can support your student, when they are at school.

18

Frequently asked questions

Students in high school and university have similar questions about applying to and getting into medical school. I have tried to capture some of the most frequent questions here, along with suggestions about how to pursue answers. Note that I say *pursue answers*: this is so that you end up with the most current and accurate information, which can only come from the ultimate source. The ultimate source of information is always each medical school in the year you plan to apply.

Do medical schools favour applicants from their own universities?

Some high school students, wondering about choosing a university, think about this: Would it be better to accept an offer at a university that has a medical school they might want to attend? It is true that students from universities with medical schools make up a higher proportion of the student population at medical schools, but this does not mean that medical schools "favour" graduates from those universities. In my view, a more reasonable explanation is that *more* graduates from those universities are inclined to apply to medical school in the first place, which increases the odds that *more* of them will be accepted. What makes them more inclined? Possibly a general interest in health-care careers, which lands them in health-sciences programs, which lands them in universities that offer a wide array of undergraduate and graduate degrees related to health sciences, which tend to be universities with medical schools.

As I think it through, it also makes sense that medical-schools admission personnel might have more familiarity with programs at the university affiliated with their medical school, which could, perhaps, confer some sort of advantage on students applying from that university.

Given the large number of applicants, though, I wonder how much attention medical schools give to the university an applicant has attended. I can't speak for medical schools: it's possible they give this lots of attention, and also possible they give it very little.

One possible advantage to attending a university that has a medical school is that it may be easier for you to connect with medical students, through clubs and groups on campus. If you think this might be helpful for you, then that might factor into your decision about universities.

Not every medical school publishes statistics about the source universities of their applicants, but you might get some information from the Association of Faculties of Medicine of Canada, which produces a variety of statistics about medical-school students on a regular basis. But don't be discouraged if you if you are planning to attend a university without a medical school, since those students get in as well.

Should I choose an "easier" degree program to get better grades?

Since it could be argued that excellent grades are a key part of gaining admission to medical school, many students wonder if it might be better to choose a so-called "easier" degree program, to help them fare well academically. I frequently hear students protest, "But, my degree program is really hard, don't they know that a B in my discipline is really an A is another discipline?"

Maybe. But, they might also be too busy to notice that kind of detail about every type of degree they see (often more than 100 in an applicant pool) from every university in Canada (which has more than ninety universities).

I encourage prospective medical-school applicants to consider their academic path carefully. For example, the career counsellor in me generally celebrates exploring a variety of disciplines during university to get a sense of what you really love doing and are good at. However, if you are thinking about medical school, I urge caution. This is because medical schools assess cumulative GPA, and a couple of courses where your grades are less than stellar might compromise your competitiveness for medical school. That's not to say that if you explore an interesting course or two during your program that you will necessarily get lower grades, or that you can't apply to medical school if you do get a few lower grades. You know yourself best, so this is simply a moment to pause and think before making decisions.

Will being at a "better" university help?

Canada has many universities, and no medical schools "rank" them or indicate how attending one or another will affect your application. If I'm reviewing 12,000 applications, and I'm ordering them to identify the top 300 GPAs, will I even care (or have time to notice) what university each GPA is from?

Maybe. Maybe not. Only a medical school can answer that question (if it will).

It seems logical to me that, depending on a university's programs and population, that certain universities might have more students inclined toward medical school in the first place. For example, universities with large and robust health sciences programs might, as a matter of course, have more students thinking about medical school. This doesn't mean that the university is necessarily "better," but it might mean that it's a better (or worse) environment for you. Think about what helps you learn, what kind of community you feel best in, and whether you prefer competitive environments or collaborative environments. This can help you make a uniquely personal decision about which university is "better" (for you).

I also encourage you to examine some of the institutional branding and marketing that universities use to promote themselves. Universities are businesses, and need to attract students, tuition, and research dollars to stay alive and grow. What they say about themselves does not necessarily reflect what others think about them, or convey the entire picture. Does this messaging stand up to a broader audience?

Maybe it does and maybe it doesn't. Only you can decide.

Will impressive extracurricular activities offset lower academic scores?

Generally speaking, your work, volunteering, extracurricular activities, awards, and other experiences form a major part of your application to medical school. The question to consider in medical-school applications (or to ask a medical school directly) might be, "At what point in the process do you review my activities? (Is it at the same time as my GPA and/or MCAT score, or later?)" Note that the answer to this question might depend on whether you are an undergraduate or graduate student.

If a medical school will answer *this* question, you can figure out the answer to your *other* question (at least in the context of that medical school). For example, if a medical school responds that it reviews your activities at the same time as your GPA and/or MCAT score, then you could hope that your activities might mitigate a lower GPA or MCAT score. If it responds that it reviews your activities after it looks at your GPA and/or MCAT score, then you would have little reason to hope that your activities might mitigate a lower GPA or MCAT score.

The other way to answer this question is to apply and see what happens. You might get specific feedback about where your application didn't meet the applicant-pool standard for that year.

It's important to be realistic, but it's also helpful to note that, in my experience, there are exceptions to every rule. I know students who, on paper, didn't look like very competitive candidates. Yet, they got accepted. I know other students who seemed very similar to these students—not that competitive on paper—and didn't get accepted. Sometimes, it's difficult to predict what will happen.

Be careful about letting anyone discourage or encourage you in the application process, unless that input is coming from the medical schools themselves. Only medical schools decide who gets into medical schools—not guidance counsellors, parents, advisors, or current medical students.

> **INSIDER INSIGHT**
> I believe that the most successful approach to gaining admission to medical school involves a combination of realism and persistence.

Is it better to do more undergraduate courses or go to graduate school?

I define "better" as "better" for you, and that will vary from student to student. Having said that, medical schools do seem to place priority on undergraduate grades at the moment. If your undergraduate grades seem like a stumbling block in your application, you may be considering whether to take more undergraduate courses to boost your cumulative GPA.

As you make that decision, consider these questions:

- Is there a way to take more undergraduate courses that will do double duty? (Think about finishing off a minor, or getting knowledge in a new subject area, or connecting with additional career options.)

- Are you interested in graduate school already? (If so, it might make more sense to pursue graduate school. Think about whether you have a topic you'd like to study in depth, whether you have a graduate-school opportunity available, and whether you want to get an advanced degree.)

- Have you checked with medical schools about how either of these options would affect your GPA, from their perspective? From their perspective, what are the pros and cons of more undergraduate courses? What are the pros and cons of a graduate degree?

What are your questions?

You likely have other questions not covered here. I encourage you to pursue information that will help you make decisions that are right for you and for your situation. What is "right" may change from year to year. My major caution is allowing others to "answer" questions for you, without scrutinizing the source of their information. If you are asking specific questions about processes (e.g., "Is lifeguarding considered a 'leadership' activity?"), you need to get the answers from the medical schools to which you apply in the year you apply. If you are asking questions about people's experiences (e.g., "What did you wish you had known when you applied?"), then, of course, you can consult friends, family members, and others.

Where can you find answers?

As mentioned many times in this book, always go to the source for information. Who are the people or organizations that will make the decisions? They are the source. Here are three options that you may find useful as you seek answers to your questions:

- the Ontario Medical School Application Service (OMSAS), for medical-school application processes in Ontario
- medical-school admissions staff at medical schools across Canada
- the Association of Faculties of Medicine of Canada, for connection to all medical schools in Canada, and for reports and statistics about medical students, medical-school programming, and residencies

19

Applying outside Canada

If you are applying to medical school, you likely know about the option of applying outside Canada.

A medical-school recruitment officer from a foreign medical school has told me that his program really loves Canadian applicants because they are such strong students and do so well. He attributes this to the highly competitive nature of getting into medical school in Canada, noting that students who "only just" miss getting an offer in Canada often apply to his program. These students are not "bad" students, by any stretch. They are excellent candidates.

Depending on your situation, a medical school outside Canada can be an option worth investigating. Be cautious, however, about the status of foreign medical credentials in Canada. Many students who take their MD abroad hope to return to Canada to practise, and foreign medical schools might say this is easy—but that's not the current reality.

Programs in the United States

Among graduates from foreign medical schools, graduates from US medical schools seem to have the easiest time returning to Canada to practise.

It helps that, when you apply to residency programs at the end of your medical school degree, the Canadian Residency Match Service (CaRMS) appears to treat Canadian and US students the same way. As far as I can tell, students at Canadian schools can apply to the US match process, and students at US schools can apply to the Canadian match process. I encourage you to consult the CaRMS website for the most up-to-date information, before you choose a US medical school.

The US has two types of programs that confer medical degrees: allopathic programs confer the degree doctor of medicine (MD), and osteopathic programs confer the degree doctor of osteopathy (DO). Graduates from DO programs are considered international medical graduates (IMGs) when they apply to practise in Canada, so this is something to carefully note.

If you are not competitive for a Canadian medical school, you will likely not be competitive for a top-tiered US allopathic medical school, either. It's possible that not being at one of these schools might affect your residency competitiveness at the end of your MD. Check the CaRMS website to find out more.

As someone who used to coordinate the hiring of physicians, I believe that the least complicated time to return to Canada is between your MD and residency training, if you want to practise in Canada. That is, rather than completing your MD and residency in the US, you would complete your MD in the US and your residency in Canada. By completing your residency in Canada, your ultimate licensing is Canadian, and it therefore makes it much easier to hire you in Canada.

Completing your MD and residency in the US can be a good option, especially if you want to work in the US. It's possible, however, that you may face disadvantages as a Canadian student applying to residency programs in the US. For example, when you apply to a US residency program as a non-US citizen, are you on equal footing with your American classmates? If a residency program is extremely small, desirable, or competitive, the seemingly inconsequential issues of citizenship might factor into acceptance decisions. (Who is easier to choose—the one who needs extra paperwork to work in the US, or the one who doesn't?)

Programs in the Caribbean, Europe, and Australia

Attracting Canadian students is big business for foreign medical schools these days. The Caribbean has more than fifty medical schools, and Europe (notably Ireland) and Australia have many more.

One of these schools might be a good option for you, if you want to work as a doctor in the country where you get your MD.

If you answered yes to these questions, you may be ready to apply to an international medical school.

Be sure to investigate the residency-program options of the school you plan to attend. For example, if you attend a Caribbean school, you must complete your residency in the United States. How might attending a Caribbean school affect your competitiveness with students from US schools, especially if you are a non-US citizen?

> **ASK YOURSELF**
>
> Where do I want to live and work as a doctor? (Or perhaps, Do I want to return to a country where I have roots?)
>
> Do I understand the risks for getting into a Canadian residency program as someone attending a foreign school?
>
> Do I understand the cost difference between attending medical school in Canada versus outside Canada?
>
> Do I understand the implications of applying to residency programs in another country as a Canadian student?

Risks and rewards of taking your MD abroad

I worry whether students applying abroad are fully informed about the ramifications of studying abroad. Most of the students I see think they will automatically be able to come back to Canada to practise.

Remember that licensure in Canada involves three steps: completing an MD, completing residency training, and passing licensing exams. These steps can become onerous for people with non-Canadian qualifications.

If you are considering a foreign medical school and want to return to Canada, check the website of the World Directory of Medical Schools. It has a list of schools that are approved by the Medical Council of Canada (the organization that licenses physicians to practise in Canada).

If a school is on that list, Canada may recognize the credentials of its graduates. If a school is **not** on the list, though, it means Canada most certainly will **not** recognize the credentials of its graduates.

Note the term *may* in the recognition of credentials from schools on the list. There's no guarantee.

I know many foreign-trained doctors from other countries, who graduated from medical schools that are acknowledged by the Medical Council of Canada. They still face a long and difficult road to practising medicine in Canada. I have a friend who practised pediatric oncology in Germany for nearly twenty years, before marrying a Canadian. Despite his extensive experience in a westernized health-care system, he is now going through the following steps to practise in Canada: writing expensive exams, repeating his entire pediatric residency (four years), and completing further fellowships (at least one more year).

You may understand, based on this example, why I recommend trying to get back to Canada between an MD and residency training, rather than waiting until you are fully licensed in another country. If you return after you complete both your MD and residency in another country, you are considered a "foreign-trained doctor," like my friend. If you can avoid that difficult label, I recommend it: at the moment, it's very challenging, expensive, and time-consuming to get relicensed in Canada.

Foreign medical schools might try to reassure you by saying something like "Canadian graduates from our program apply to Canadian residency programs, just like their counterparts in Canada." Technically, this is true, and schools sometimes back up this kind of statement with a success

INSIDER INSIGHT
Statistics out of CaRMS vary some from year to year, but generally show low match rates (e.g., 1% to 3%) for international medical graduates applying for residency spots in Canada.

story from a graduate. But, a more frank statement would describe the difficulty of returning to Canada for training or to practise. At the current time, yes, you can apply along with your Canadian counterparts, **but** it is rare to be successful. Most Canadian students attending foreign medical schools will **not** be able to get into a Canadian residency program. That's hard news to hear, I'm sure, when you feel desperate to "get in somewhere." It's important news, though: you are vulnerable, and need to think carefully and critically about the ramifications of a foreign MD program.

In 2018 in Canada, more than a hundred students from Canadian medical schools did not match to a residency spot.[1] It makes sense that the odds of a match get more challenging if you are applying from a medical school outside Canada.

Consult the CaRMS R-1 match results (for first-year residency spots) on the CaRMS website for more information.

ASK YOURSELF

If you are considering a foreign medical school, does it offer coaching for residency applications? If it does, how well does it know the requirements of the Canadian residency-application process?

You may not know that students attending Canadian medical schools get coaching from their programs to help them apply for residency. I have done this coaching myself for years, working with fourth-year medical students on preparing CVs, personal letters, references, and interviews, which are all required elements of the residency-application process.

Foreign medical training, however, can deliver much (or all) of what you want. You can become a doctor and practise medicine, although maybe (probably) not in Canada. (For example, most Canadian students studying at Caribbean schools end up practising in the United States.) Not coming back to Canada is not a good or bad thing—it is simply something to consider as you make your choices.

How to avoid timeline agony

If you opt to apply to a foreign medical school because you don't think Canadian schools will accept you, be careful about timelines.

INSIDER INSIGHT

My observation is that Canadian applicants to foreign schools tend to be strong candidates and have a high likelihood of being accepted.

I've spoken with many students tormented because they've received an acceptance to a foreign medical school (many foreign schools have three intakes per year) before they know if they have been accepted in Canada. Putting down a deposit to confirm your spot somewhere that is actually your second choice (and possibly a risky choice, depending on your goals) can be extremely difficult when you don't know whether your first choice will come through. Many students (especially those who ultimately want to practise in Canada) choose to apply to foreign medical schools after Canadian programs have rejected them.

Note

1. "CFMS Strongly Urges Government of Canada to Provide Sustainable Solutions to Canadian Medical Graduates Unable to Secure a Residency Training Position," Canadian Federation of Medical Students, published May 29, 2018, accessed July 5, 2018, https://www.cfms.org/news/2018/05/29/press-release-cfms-strongly-urges.html.

20

How to be happy with your outcomes

One of my favourite times of year is May—the time when I get lots of email and phone calls and visits from students who are ecstatic to report they have succeeded in their application to medical school.

I also hear from students at this time of year who are disappointed. I am always heartened when they are not beaten by that disappointment, although they feel it acutely. I love it when they tell me that getting help has allowed them to feel that they put their best foot forward, and that they know where to go from here. That doesn't mean they don't face some sadness or loss of confidence, or or that they don't need time to regroup. But they have enough support and information to move forward—to a possible future application and to other options.

ASK YOURSELF

If you are lucky enough to receive more than one offer and need to make decisions, try narrowing down your options with these questions:

Where would I like to live during the next three to four years?

What school culture and learning style seems to fit me best? Have I got enough information to make a decision about that?

What are the residency-match statistics from each medical school? (Do their graduates get the residencies they want?)

If you have been successful in your application this time, I congratulate you! This is a major life accomplishment and you should feel justifiably relieved, proud, and happy. You might even feel a little guilty, if you have friends who weren't as fortunate.

No matter where you go, your medical school years will likely lead you to strong growth and lasting friendships. Congratulations, again!

If this wasn't your year, I feel your disappointment and encourage you to remember that **rejection is normal**: it does not make you a failure (no

> **INSIDER INSIGHT**
> Check out chapter 16 for strategies and ideas about where to go from here.

matter what that nasty voice inside your head may say). Of course, this may not help you feel better in this moment. I encourage you to get support from those who love you and remember that the path is not yet finished. It continues and you only have to step back on it and keep moving forward.

It can be stressful

Managing alternate plans

Many graduating students are particularly stressed at this time of year because they are balancing a couple of options at the same time. They didn't know if they would get into medical school, so many have put backup plans in motion, such as applications for jobs or master's programs. Or they need to start putting those plans in motion. They don't find out about their medical-school results until May or even later, so sometimes they have already commenced a backup plan by the time they find out. Then, they are faced with decisions: Should I leave what I'm doing and start medical school in September? Should I stay where I am and apply again later? How do I tell my supervisor that I need to quit? If I've been wait-listed, how will I find a place to live in time?

In these cases, there is a lot of uncertainty. And a lot of waiting. Most of us aren't particularly good at managing uncertainty and waiting. It can feel pretty stressful as you dangle in the middle of several possible options, not knowing what will happen next. This can be especially true if you find yourself in this situation after completing a degree, because everyone tends to ask you, "What are you doing next?" It can become an annoying question, when you just don't have the answers yet.

Some students choose to take a summer job, so they can leave "naturally" at the end of it, if they suddenly get off a wait list and get accepted to medical school. Others start a full-time job and simply give notice, if they are accepted to medical school. Most graduate programs and supervisors will be disappointed, but not shocked, if you have to leave because of an offer to medical school: they are aware that it's a rare opportunity that can't easily be deferred.

My general advice is this: do your best to be kind and ethical if acceptance to medical school means you have to leave something you've started. Remember that people appreciate time to make plans to replace you (whether you've started an education program or a job). If you help make the transition as easy on people as you can, they will usually be very happy for your turn of events.

Seeking help

If you are trying to make decisions about which medical school to choose, or what to do because you weren't accepted, I encourage you to connect with your support system and others who can help you.

For decisions about backup plans and reapplication strategies, you might talk to parents, family, and friends; guidance counsellors in high school, or career centres at universities; and academic advisors, and undergraduate chairs or assistants at universities. And consult chapter 3 in this resource: it has ideas about ways to explore career options, including books and other websites.

For application and interview strategies, and help with preparation, consider parents, family, and friends; guidance counsellors in high school or career centres at universities; and writing centres at universities.

For decisions about choosing schools, you can learn a lot by seeking out organizations and licensing bodies where doctors communicate with each other and the world. Here are some examples of organizations:

- Canadian Medical Association (CMA) and provincial counterparts—e.g., Ontario Medical Association (OMA), Alberta Medical Association (AMA), New Brunswick Medical Society (NBMS), Doctors of BC, and so on
- Royal College of Physicians and Surgeons of Canada (RCPSC)
- Medical Council of Canada (MCC)
- Association of Faculties of Medicine of Canada (AFMC)

- Canadian Residency Match Service (CaRMS)

Many students seek coaching from their high school guidance office or university career centre (usually at no cost), or from a private medical-careers specialist (fee for service). These people can be helpful with strategy, thinking through options, application review, interview practice, and more.

Clarify your goals, clarify your options

Students who know why they are applying to medical school (not just because it seems like the next logical step, or because it's what "smart" students do), and know what other careers might suit them, tend to end up in good places. This is true whether they eventually end up in medical school or choose another path.

Whatever your next steps, I encourage you to keep moving. Students who stagnate in a cycle of medical-school applications, and don't move forward with other career options between applications, seem to suffer most. I worked with a student who was the third person in her family to pursue medical school. She was extremely stressed: her two older brothers had applied to medical school and had been unsuccessful. This was part of the problem, but not the main problem. No, the main problem was that her brothers were unwilling to consider anything else and, in her words, "live in my parent's house even though they are approaching thirty years old and do nothing but play video games all day." Yikes. I wish I could have helped her brothers (and parents) in some way.

Every year, I meet with students who have moved on to other "in between" options while they wait to reapply to medical school, and wind up discovering that they really love where they've ended up. Whether it's in other clinical professions (nursing, physical therapy, medical social work), nonclinical roles in the hospital environment (hospital administration, medical geneticist, physician recruiter), community health settings (community support worker, education coordinator, health educator), or scientific settings (research assistant, clinical trials administrator, lab technologist), people find their place in the health sector—or outside it. Many times, students opt not to reapply to medical school because they have found a great career. Sometimes, experience with other career options serves to remotivate students for the next round of applications, because they have gained even more clarity that *physician* is the role they aspire to most.

I hope that if you become a physician, your career is all you dreamed it would be. Happily, you can find career satisfaction, productivity, and success no matter where you end up. I know this from my two decades of working with students. I also know that keeping a positive attitude and open mind about next steps can be key to finding that path and enjoying it, once you are on it.

Whatever your story, whatever your journey, I wish you the very best and hope that this resource contributes to your success.

I will be cheering for you.

ABOUT THE AUTHOR

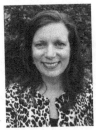

Christine Fader has extensive experience as a coach for students applying to medical school. She has worked as a career counsellor for the last twenty years, at Queen's University and in private practice. Her experience also includes eight years volunteering on a medical-school admissions committee. She has worked with thousands of students through her highly successful workshops on how to prepare applications and interviews for medical school and residency training.